Dear Dr. Jock...
The People's Guide to
Sports and Fitness

Dear Dr. Jock...
The People's Guide to

David C. Bachman, M.D., and
Marilynn Preston

Illustrations by Joe DeVelasco

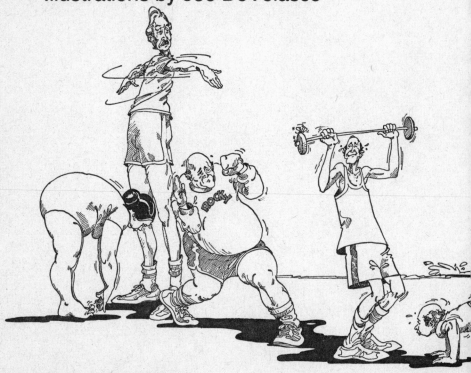

A Dutton Paperback
E. P. Dutton   New York

Sports and Fitness

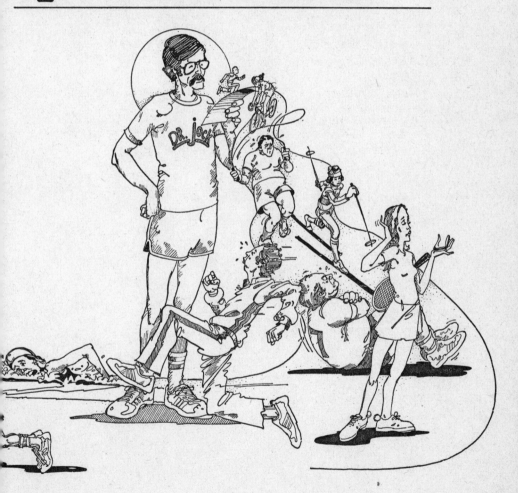

For information contact:

E. P. Dutton, 2 Park Avenue, New York, N.Y. 10016

Library of Congress Cataloging in Publication Data
Bachman, David C.   The Dr. Jock book.
1. Sports medicine. I. Preston, Marilynn, joint author. II. Title.
RC1210.B26 1980   617′.1027   79-17772

ISBN: 0-525-93066-3

Published simultaneously in Canada by
Clarke, Irwin & Company Limited, Toronto and Vancouver

Designed by Mary Beth Bosco

10 9 8 7 6 5 4 3 2 1

First Edition

This book is dedicated to all the people who refuse to take Robert Maynard Hutchins's exercise advice lying down

Contents

Acknowledgments

Knowledge grows like coral. It is living, ever-changing, always building—the accretion of many bits and pieces of information.

This book evolved from reading and talking and listening to many different people—to experts, friends, acquaintances, mates, parents, patients, editors and all those concerned others who have taken the time to write Dr. Jock.

We should single out Gloria Scoby for her energy and enthusiasm and Mike Argirion for his early support. Drue Cass did the serious typing, Connie Schrader and Amy Clampitt did the final editing and Joe DeVelasco helped it all hang together with his wonderful illustrations.

Without all of them and all of you, there wouldn't be any of this. Thanks.

I. Get Hooked

1. Dr. Jock–

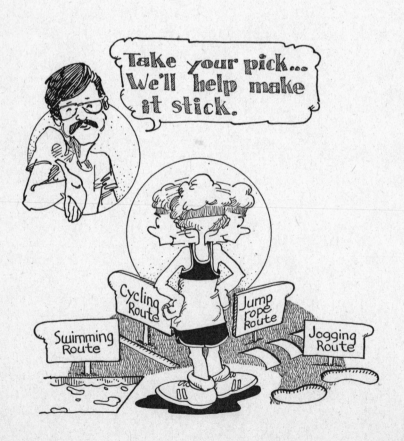

The People's Coach

Dear Dr. Jock:

My husband has a torn rotator cuff and finds it painful to play golf. He is 72 years old and has had this condition for eight years. Is there anything he can do for this? Is surgery guaranteed? Exercises? Can 72-year-old muscles regenerate?

R.K., Beverly Hills, California

Dear Dr. Jock:

Can you recommend any exercises or weight training to help relieve shin splints? Thank you.

I.L., Miami Beach, Florida

Dear Dr. Jock:

I'd like to improve my "mental" performance in basketball games. How does psychology affect performance? Also, under pressure I always seem to fold. How "mentally" can I help myself with this pressure? Do you have any other comments, suggestions or ideas on how to improve mental performance? Thanks.

D.K., Andover, Massachusetts

P.S. This is for myself and also to aid in my school project. Please print in "Sports Plus" as soon as possible.

Letters. We get letters. We get sacks and stacks of letters from people all over the country, from uptown Manhattan to Route 2 in Bulls Gap, Tennessee. We get letters from runners, walkers, hikers, rope jumpers, cyclists, swimmers, tennis players and other recreational athletes who—just like you—are working on their fitness, or wanting to.

We're not talking about the pros. We're not talking about the big-time athletes with coaches of their own, or those precious few superstar jocks whose molten steel physiques have been biomechanically analyzed up one fast-twitch fiber and down the other.

We're talking about garden-variety folks just like you, players of all persuasions who want to slim down, tighten up, boost cardiovascular endurance, sweat off some of the inevitable pressures of everyday life and, in the process, have as much fun as possible.

We're talking about the healthy, active biology teacher from Ft. Lauderdale who wrote Dr. Jock the day she finally huffed and puffed her way to 5 full miles without stopping. She was hooked, she admitted, and wanted to know if 63 was too old to begin training for a marathon. (It's not, if you take it slow and easy.)

We're talking about the men's B tennis player from Sepulveda who had dumbbells and some exercises to prevent tennis elbow but didn't know how much or how many or how often.

We're talking about the lady with the baby in a Phoenix suburb who doesn't have the free time or extra money to join an expensive health club but is desperate to do something about the jelly-roll blues hanging off her hips and thighs.

In short, we're talking about citizen athletes like you, who don't know where to turn for the latest information on sports medicine. What is fitness anyway? Is it better to run fast for a short distance or longer and farther? What's the best way to prevent tennis elbow? Why are warm-ups the first line of defense in avoiding more than 60 percent of all sports injuries? What about nutrition: are there special high energy foods, drinks, vitamins and supplements that will spark a championship performance?

If you're on a regular exercise program now, or are ashamed about how many you've dropped out of, you need to understand the answers to all those questions, and more. You need to know why pushing yourself too hard, too fast, is the worst thing you can do in exercise. You need to know about strength and flexibility and how best to develop the kind of body awareness that brings your mind into play.

You need information, guidance, assurance and you need it fast because if you don't know what you're doing when you're doing something strenuous, you're going to get hurt. Millions of recreational athletes do every year, and the problem is getting worse. And painfully expensive.

And that's where Dr. Jock comes in. Three years ago, we started a newspaper column in the *Chicago Tribune* geared to answering your questions about the aches, pains, fears, follies and medical myths that can get in the way of you and your sweaty good time.

Now Dr. Jock is a nationally syndicated Q & A column, a friendly collaboration between two professionals—a doctor and a writer—who know what a tough struggle it can be to get hooked on regular exercise and who want to make it safer and more enjoyable for you.

David Bachman is a medical doctor, an orthopedic surgeon who specializes in treating athletes and sports injuries. Marilynn Preston is a Chicago journalist who conceived of Dr. Jock. When pressed for medical credentials, she says she specializes in avoiding sports injuries—always her own. David has been team doc for both the Bulls and the Hustle—the men's and women's pro basketball teams in Chicago—as well as director of the Center for Sports Medicine at Northwestern University Medical School.

Together, as Dr. Jock, we field all kinds of urgent inquiries and heartfelt pleas: "Help! I'm fat and 40 and I've failed at running 3 different times—is exercycling just as good?" Or: "My daughter is 12 and a swimmer. If I let her lift weights will she get boys' shoulders?"

We get cards and letters and plaintive cries from athletes all over the country who are concerned about their fitness and eager for sensible information that will help them get through some miserably painful episodes. We've heard from Little Leaguers with sore arms, and junior executives with stiff backs and there was one lovely lady from the Southwest who told us she totally turned her life around when she took up tennis at the age of 71. (She wanted to know if she could play without a bra.)

And in letter after angry, frustrated letter, we've heard from runners who have tried 4 kinds of running shoes, 2 orthotics, castor oil, elastic bandages, vitamin E, plus all 10 sessions of rolfing—and still can't get over their knee pain. Usually, about 6 or 7 different treatments down the line, they are curious about acupuncture.

And why not? When you're trying to get fit, you'll try anything to keep going. You've got to keep going. It doesn't matter who you are, at what age you begin, or how quickly you move from one level of play to the next: the key to getting fit is to keep going.

The Dr. Jock column, and this book, are designed to keep you going. No matter your age, or sex, or sport, no matter if you are the best woman on the town rugby team or the slowest runner on your block, you can learn to play better, enjoy your sport more and—most important of all—keep from injuring yourself. We won't make you into an Olympic champion but we can help you become the best athlete you can be.

George Leonard, social critic, author and president of the Association for Humanistic Psychology, wrote a powerful book several years ago called *The Ultimate Athlete*. As defined by Leonard, the Ultimate Athlete is "the one who joins mind, body and spirit in the dance of existence . . . who explores the inner and outer being . . . who plays the larger game, The Game of Games, with full awareness, aware of life and death and willing to accept the pain and joy that awareness brings . . ."

We're none of us quite there yet. If you're like most people in the country, your inner being and your outer being are only beginning to touch. You're still too worried about your EKG to care much about your ESP. You may, indeed, be longing to float and fly and feel weightless, but chances are your workouts are still dogged by blisters, stitches and burning blasts of knee pain. Maybe you've already experienced one of those peak moments that athletes feel when they are performing in perfect harmony, or maybe you're still too involved with your respiration to give much thought to your inspiration. That's okay too, for now. Don't be in too big a hurry. The important thing is you're moving in the right direction—toward fitness, health, wellness and self-care and away from sickness, sloth, junk food and banana cream pies.

This book will help you emerge, as we introduce you to a philosophy of fitness that offers pleasure and satisfaction along the way. As you run, swim, jump and cycle yourself into condition—as you keep going—you'll feel the burden of your everyday stress and strain begin to lift. Problems won't disappear, but you will find them more manageable. You'll feel stronger, more energetic, more able to cope with nasty salesclerks, broken cars, neurotic housemates, bureaucratic bunglings and the rest of life's stress-inducing irritations.

It's the theme throughout this book that the fitter you feel, the better your life will be. Once you're really hooked on fitness, your body will change shape. Your muscles will tone up, your waistline will return and you can hope that the cottage cheese collecting at the back of your thighs will vanish forever. As your body slims down, your mind will expand, people who haven't seen you in months will admire your cheekbones and notice your sense of calm and ask you how you did it. They may be too envious, really, to hear your answer, but we bet you'll love telling them anyway.

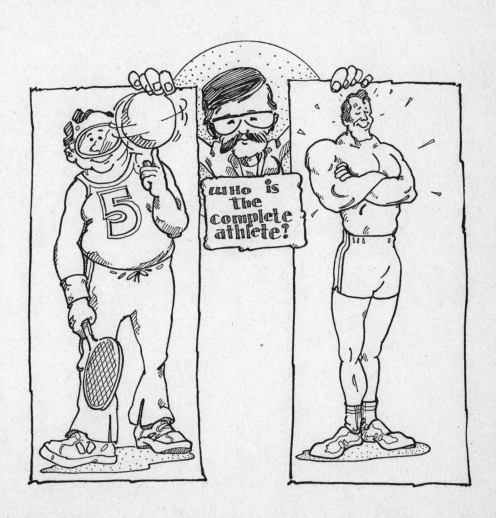

2. Self-Care Is the

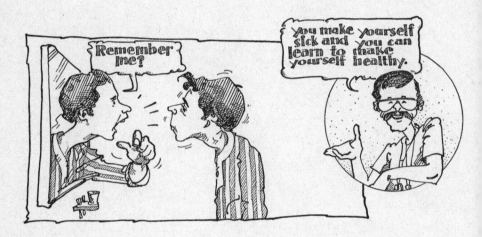

Best Care

Dear Dr. Jock:

I'm a 13-year-old girl. I weigh 120 pounds and I'm only 5'1". My thighs are flabby and they melt right into my knees. Will riding a stationary bicycle help me trim off this ugly fat?

D.S.R., Arcadia, California

Dear Dr. Jock:

I have been practicing yoga exercises for 22 years and doing over 30 different positions, including headstands for 10-12 minutes and also 30-35 full push-ups (raising my pulse to 110 or better). I used to exercise every day for 50 minutes but now only 4 times a week. My diet is very balanced, I have never taken a vitamin pill, do not smoke or drink, and have always maintained my excellent physical condition. I will be 81 years young in a few months, and I believe my program has slowed my aging. My wife says it's longevity genes in the family. What is your opinion?

H.W., Coral Gables, Florida

Dear Dr. Jock:

Five months ago I developed what the doctors call tendinitis. The first doctor I went to took X-rays and gave me cortisone shots and after two treatments said it was bursitis or rheumatism and said I should rest my arm and not do any exercise of any kind. After not using my right arm to avoid the pain in my shoulder for six weeks, it did not get any better. I then went to a different doctor who did exactly what the first one did (only he charged $30 more!). After my second shot he told me that it was a chronic condition and that I would have to learn to live with it. It's been five months and I still get pain in my right shoulder and I used to enjoy a game of golf every now and then but now I can't even play that. I'm getting very depressed. Can you advise me on this?

M.F., Des Moines, Iowa

All recreational athletes have one thing in common—they want to keep going. If you're not hooked on fitness yet, you want to be. And you know that getting hooked isn't always a piece of cake. Indeed, it may mean denying yourself that piece of cake in favor of an apple and twenty-three raisins. But you want to keep going all the same. You are concerned about being the best athlete you can be with the fewest possible aches and pains. You are concerned about your health, your general well-being, your family.

In this chapter we're concerned with one of the underlying principles of a growing movement in sports medicine—that you, the runner, the cyclist, the tennis player, the patient, must understand your own role in keeping healthy. Doctors can tell you the best fitness plan, but the success and failure of that plan depends on you. So does injury prevention. So does knowing how to take care of some of those minor aches and bruises. So does understanding how your body works so you won't overuse it, and get sick as a result. In other words, you are responsible for your own health.

Taking responsibility for your own health is important for several reasons. One is pure economics. Right now, medical costs in this country are skyrocketing and if you think that last $60 visit to the emergency room was outrageous ("But the doctor didn't even spend three minutes with me! And it turns out there was nothing wrong anyway!"), think of what $200 billion worth of visits, tests, X-rays and labor costs are doing to the inflation picture.

Think for a minute about how much it cost you and your family to get sick last year. About how much you paid every week, or every month, to a third-party insurer. How good was the medical care, anyhow? If you had something dramatic, like a kidney transplant or a heart bypass, it will have been very good. But what about niggling backache, shoulder pains, ankle sprains and knee strains—those treatments that nickle-and-dime you to death and still don't get rid of your problem?

Injuries are costly, and they rob you of your peace of mind, your dignity. You feel helpless and frustrated. The more we have to depend on expensive hospital care and busy specialists, the more time we waste on unnecessary doctor visits and unnecessary surgeries, the greater the nation's health bill . . . and the worse we feel. It's a vicious cycle and one way to break it before it breaks us is to get more people involved in fitness and self-care. We have to educate all the millions of health users, and abusers too, that there are safe, reasonable alternatives available. We have to teach people that in the long run the best care is self-care: exercising regularly, eating less junk, reducing stress, body awareness, etc. And the first step in learning to take better care of yourself is to accept the notion that you are responsible for your own health.

At the base of all the self-care, self-healing, holistic philosophies that have sprung up throughout the country is the medical truism that, in more cases than we'd like to believe, you make yourself sick. *Why* you do it isn't the issue here: the important thing is to accept that you do it. You make yourself sick and you can learn to make yourself healthy—it's your choice, your responsibility. You have the ability to heal yourself, to take care of yourself, to develop your fitness so that you are less susceptible to heart attacks, strokes, high blood pressure, depression.

That doesn't mean you should cancel next Tuesday's appointment about your chronic backache, or drop your Blue Cross policy and decide to go it alone on pure faith and a resting pulse of 42. Nor are we recommending that busloads of recreational athletes make regular runs to Lourdes—though don't doubt that some aching runners would gladly go. No, as in getting fit, you have to rely on common sense, and go slowly. To understand the basics of self-care takes time and study.

But you are ready to make time for understanding the principles of health and fitness. You know, deep down, in your vascularly-improved heart of hearts that the more self-sufficient you are when it comes to understanding and using your body, the better runner, skier, tennis player, mate, lover, worker, boss, parent you'll be.

Your doctor may be one of the greatest in the profession, but if you're not doing something on your own to keep your heart and lungs strong, your blood pressure down, your fitness level up and your muscles toned and flexible, *you* are going to suffer. And if you suffer, there goes your tennis game, your 10-mile daily run, your M-W-F racquetball game, not to mention, on occasion, your life.

THERE'S NOTHING NEW ABOUT SELF-CARE

So, when we're talking about self-care or holistic health we're not really talking about anything crazy or drastic, or even anything new. The basics have been around for centuries. Indeed, the common-sense, self-care, take-responsibility-for-your-own-health movement was very strong in this country for a while during the 19th century, B.O.M. (Before Organized Medicine). In those days every family had its home health guide. One of the most popular was *Domestic Medicine*, published in 1830. Its author, Dr. John C. Gunn, was one of those rare health professionals with a real interest in demystifying medicine, even though his livelihood depended on taking care of other people. The so-called learned men, Gunn said, used fancy medical terms "to conceal the naked poverty and bareness of the sciences. If the great mass of the people knew how much pains were taken by scientific men to throw dust in their eyes by the use of ridiculous and high-sounding terms, mankind would soon be undeceived as to the little difference that really exists between themselves and the very learned portion of the community." We hope this book will help clear some of that dust away.

TWENTY MILLION SPORTS INJURIES—MOST OF THEM PREVENTABLE

We will tell you what you need to know to prevent most injuries, and help you distinguish between injuries you can care for yourself and those that you ought to see a doctor about. Sometimes, seeing a doctor may be just a step you need to take to rule out the possibility of serious injury. It is no use being nagged by doubts or fears about what is really causing your aches and pains. That yellow-green bruise will heal more slowly if you go around thinking it is some new kind of cancer.

Every year, according to an oft-repeated figure, more than twenty million people twist an ankle, strain a tendon, pull a muscle or wrench a back, and are treated for such sports-related injuries. We have no way of knowing whether the figure is accurate or not. If we were betting, we would guess it's probably on the low side. Undoubtedly there are millions more would-be athletes who injure themselves early in the game, not badly enough to see a doctor but enough to scare them away from regular exercise.

This book is geared to keeping you going. That's the only trick to fitness—you have to keep going. The best way to do that is to prevent and avoid injuries. The next best is to learn a little basic first aid so that when you do get hurt, you will understand what has happened and what you should do about it. Some minor strains and sprains you can care for on your own, *should* care for on your own if you want to break the vicious cycle of doctor-patient dependency. If your injury does require a doctor's care, the more you know about it, the better your treatment will be. You can't make your body heal faster than it wants to, but you can avoid doing things that get in the way of healing and prolong your recovery. You can learn to use your mind to cope with body pain better. You can agree to work toward your recovery in a positive way, instead of getting upset or giving in to depression.

After all, doctors know a lot about how your mind and your body work, but they don't know everything. You might be surprised to hear that they probably only understand about 10 percent, maybe 5 percent, of all the things they'll eventually come to learn about how the human body operates. We progress, but we progress slowly. Painfully slow it seems at times, like now, when our heaviest guns are aimed toward finding a cure for cancer and many of our best and brightest researchers are still shooting blanks. But we seem to be moving now—again, slowly and painfully—away from the one assassin–no conspiracy theory of a viral cause for cancer and toward the idea that we are causing many of our own cancers. That it is *our* pollution, *our* chemical wastes, *our* explosions, *our* food additives, *our* industrial poisons that are cancer-causing agents in a world we created for ourselves. As a country, we will have to take responsibility for that, and act in a just and proper manner.

And as an individual, you have to take responsibility too. Your health, your ability to cope, is in *your* hands, no matter what the man from All-State would like you to believe. No one cares about you, or about your family, more than you do. Nor should they.

Yet, when push comes to shove, and we find ourselves sick or depressed or injured, we are happy to go to perfect strangers or imperfect friends—people we have been taught to believe in: the Doctors. And we are relieved to present our weak, flabby, unfit, uncared-for bodies, saying, "Cure me. My knee hurts, my back is ailing, my head aches, my tennis game is shot all to hell, and I don't really understand what's wrong but I'm sure you must . . . so cure me."

Well, if doctors were perfectly honest with their patients the first thing they'd do is ask you what you have going on in your life that is making you so sick. What are *you* doing, what are *you* feeling, what craziness is going on at the job or in the marriage that has led to your coming to see them. When doctors are perfectly honest, they will admit that in 8 out of 10 cases, the patient is doing *something*—or *not* doing something—to make himself sick. Maybe he's not dealing with stress, or is overeating himself to death. Most often, where sports injuries are involved, the cause is simply not taking the 10 minutes needed to warm up beforehand.

Most doctors aren't fools; they know where much of the responsibility for illness and injuries lies. But since most doctors aren't fools, they also know that most patients don't want responsibility, they want cures: pain relief, pills, prescriptions. They're willing to pay for anything that will keep them healthy and happy. Sorry, sports fans, but money can't buy you that.

Self-care is the best care. Like fitness, it's a life-or-death issue, and the better you know yourself and take care of yourself, the healthier and happier you'll be. The less you have to depend on busy doctors, $200-a-day hospitals, insurance companies, disability compensation or a National Health Disservice to keep you feeling strong and fit and able to cope with life's inevitable ups-and-downs (without resorting to uppers and downers), the more pleasant life is. Self-care. Do unto yourself before others can do unto you . . . and maybe do it wrong, and make you sicker. It's really very simple when you think about it.

However, getting yourself to think about how your body works, how to get it to work better, with fewer injuries, can be a struggle. "I don't understand what happened to my elbow, but it's killing me," says the tennis player who never bothered to learn the proper backhand and uses a racket with much too small a grip. Or take the runner with severe knee pain who has spent over a thousand dollars and six months looking for a cure, and who still refuses to accept that the five minutes a week he spends stretching out his leg muscles just aren't enough to keep his knee going. Understanding your sports injury and working to keep it from happening again isn't nearly as easy as getting a prescription, or taking a pill, or pleading for a shot. Too often the injured party prefers to know nothing. And hear nothing. Which is why they want everything repeated. "Doc, I've got this lousy back pain every time I swing a golf club," they say, as if sincere genuflecting will somehow make a difference. If you want to make a difference in your life, in the way you feel and look, you'll eventually have to commit yourself to self-care. That means regular exercise, better nutrition, less stress and a happier life.

Millions already have, and their numbers are growing. More and more men and women are beginning to realize that no doctor, no guru, no healer, no pain-killer, no medication is as powerful, as capable of caring and healing your body, as you are.

Self-care enthusiasts are finding each other and a lot of wonderful, medically-sound information on nutrition, exercise, stress reduction and self-healing in books and workshops and training courses all across the country. The movement is big and getting bigger. And as the word spreads, we will see more and more traditional doctors begin to shift their concern from treatment of disease to prevention, from curing disease with harsh drugs and stopgap measures to encouraging and enlightening patients to help themselves avoid disease, prevent injuries and strive toward an optimal level of wellness.

In the best of all possible worlds, that's how the developing field of sports medicine will operate. Within the bounds of traditional medicine, it will embrace some nontraditional healing concepts. Sports-medicine practitioners include orthopedic surgeons, internists, cardiologists, nutritionists, psychologists, psychiatrists, gerontologists, podiatrists and a wealth of other health professionals and paraprofessionals, all (hopefully) working to make you fully aware of the rules and regulations of preventive medicine. We want to coach our clients, our players, our partners, to be healthy and knowledgeable, not sick and weak and dependent on pills, doctors and drugs to get them through another dreary day. We would much rather educate you about the stomach-strengthening benefits of 25 bent-leg sit-ups a day than listen to another overweight businessman complain about his stress-related backache or write another prescription for Valium when we know darn well that a lot of that depression and all the Excedrin headaches between 1 and 100 would probably disappear if patients would start exercising their bodies as much as they already exercise their mouths.

In the best of all worlds, sports-medicine experts will be teaching you to *prevent* problems by reducing stress, exercising regularly, monitoring your own vital signs, eating more grains and vegetables, as well as less meat protein and fat, and deep-breathing away your problems, day by day and week after week. A journalist named Phil Weld recently spent a year on an Alicia Patterson Foundation Fellowship talking with health experts, running with New Age coaches like Dyveke Spino and George Leonard, checking in on innovative healing communities like SAGE in Berkeley, California, and Dr. John Travis's Wellness Clinic in Mill Valley, California, and Dr. Rudolph Ballentine's practice at the Himalayan Institute in Glenview, Illinois, and Honesdale, Pennsylvania. In a series of research papers, he revealed that only one half of one percent of an estimated $140 billion a year spent on health care in the country went toward health education. Forty percent of the $140 billion went to hospitals. We're not suggesting that sports-medicine experts should operate outside of hospital care, but we are hoping that they will be at the forefront of a new medicine revolution that is geared to helping you, teaching you, advising you to take better care of yourself.

SELF-CARE BEGINS WITH SELF-ANALYSIS

Self-care begins with an honest evaluation of yourself, by yourself or by some professional outfit equipped to give you a complete and expert evaluation. (See Chapter 3 for some examples.) The important thing is to be honest with yourself, and not to expect too much, too soon. You have time. You have your whole life, so be realistic about how quickly you try and change it. Go slowly and keep going—that's the trick. Don't expect yourself to run a mile your first time out. You should figure on at least one month of training for every year you've been out of condition.

The hard part, for many men especially, is to get over that old competitive drive to be the best, the first, to push until it hurts. That may have worked for you twenty years ago and it's possible that it may work for you again, but more often than not, the people who get on a regular exercise program and stick to it are people who have learned that not only isn't winning everything, it's bad for the ulcer.

The killer instinct, the competitive urge to run that other guy into the ground, is fine if it keeps you going but it probably won't. After all, how many of us can be winners all the time? The answer is *all of us can* if we simply decide to switch the rules around a little and decide that when it comes to achieving fitness, when it comes to playing sports that we enjoy and that help keep body and mind in top operating condition, *there are no losers*. You may, in fact, not win every race you enter, and you may find a tennis player that is tougher than you are or a ski slope that simply goes beyond your ability to cope, but if you do your best you can't lose.

Naturally, the same philosophy applies to women too. Just as there are no losers when it comes to getting fit, there are no reasons why women shouldn't work as hard and as long and as happily to enjoy the benefits of getting into condition. Women do, however, bring different sensitivities, different vulnerabilities, to the whole process. For one thing, women were cheated out of organized sports for a long while, and although this situation is slowly changing (thanks to the Billie Jean Kings and Title IX's of our day), we are left with whole generations of grown women who are simply unused to sports, unacquainted with regular exercise.

Needlepoint, quilting and car pools are not fitness activities, and though younger women may now be going through life feeling perfectly free and easy and even proud about running, lifting weights and beating their boyfriends at racquetball, there are great numbers of others who still have to get used to the notion that it's okay to sweat. In public. And it's okay to want to shape your body by running and by hour-long workouts in the Y pool, instead of torturing it with tight corsets, boring diets and dangerous appetite suppressants. Women are discovering that being fit will not compromise their femininity—that, in fact, getting hooked on a regular exercise program, taking 30 or 60 minutes a day, every other day, to stretch and sweat and feel revitalized, is a terrific gift they can give themselves. Once their initial fears ("Will my muscles get all ugly and bulgy like a man's if I lift weights?" or "Is it true that a regular running program will hurt my chances of getting pregnant?") turn out to be based on misinformation, women discover that to be fit means being not only stronger but also more sensitive, more responsive, and sexier. Fitness builds confidence, and confidence is at the root of femininity. The joy of sex is all wrapped up in the joy of flex.

Between 1970 and 1976 there was a whopping 400 percent increase in the number of girls participating in high school sports. Competitive women athletes are breaking records left, right and center. Things have certainly come a long way since the early 1960s, when women were still considered too fragile and too ill-equipped emotionally to be involved in sports. The two most important sports for women at Marilynn's high school—indeed, the *only* sports-related activities that were really encouraged—were ironing green gymsuits and chalking white gym shoes. It wasn't that long ago that girls who liked sports were outcasts and tomboys, who, if they didn't *let* the boy win, were thought to be seriously hampering their chances of getting married. And all that's changing too, thank goodness.

Nowadays it is quite proper, even fashionable, for women to put aside their aprons, cast off their gold chains and self-care themselves into a tummy-trimming lather by running, cycling, swimming, playing racquetball, tennis, squash and so on, just like a man. Just like a man, the female of the species is discovering that the better able she is to take care of herself, the less resentful she is when there are others who want to be taken care of.

She is also realizing that there's a right and a less-right way to get fit. Women can get ulcers and heart trouble, too—just like a man—if they're not careful to avoid pushing themselves too hard or too fast at the beginning. That means learning how to relax and breathe properly, how to warm up and get stronger in the process. It means challenging yourself enough to keep your exercise going . . . and interesting . . . but not making it so difficult that you bypass the pleasure and set yourself up for pain and failure. Regular exercise can ease menstrual cramps and stave off depression; but going about it too grimly can become a source of depression and pain. To succeed, you have to keep going: then fitness will follow naturally.

The whole process of self-care really starts rolling when you're able to look at yourself realistically. Are you a 30-year-old citizen racer looking to glean a few tips for your next cross-country ski competition? Or are you a Morton Grove mother of four who started jumping rope last week with the idea of running in the Chicago Marathon next fall? Or maybe you're a lawyer, a whiz in the criminal courts, but a fizz on the tennis courts? You've got to look at your needs, your fears, your body, your stresses, your likes and dislikes, and decide from the start that as long as you keep going at this game, you can't lose. And the secret of that is to start slowly and maintain perspective, neither looking backward at the klutz you once thought you were, nor concentrating unduly on the superstar you want to be, but paying attention to the nice person you already are.

We all have the capacity to work ourselves and our lives into shape. What we all need is to learn how to do it—how to make the workouts enjoyable as well as safe. To keep going means finding satisfaction in the process itself, not just in the finished product. What if the product never gets finished? Look at all the fun you'll have missed.

The people who get hooked on fitness have found a way to make it all fun, and you can, too. Just above Marilynn's typewriter is a quotation from a fellow named Updegraff. Accompanying it is a picture of a little country road winding through rural Vermont. The trees are at their prettiest and there's not a body in sight. The sign reads: "Happiness is found along the way, not at the end of the road." That goes for fitness, too.

3. The Ideal Do-It-

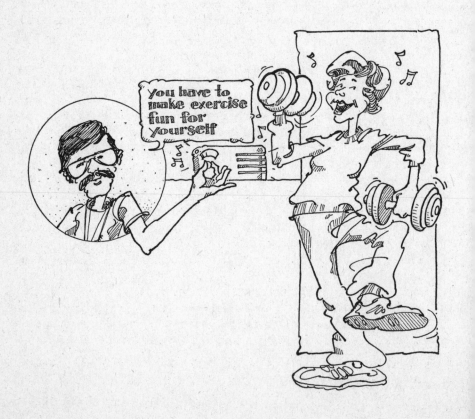

Yourself Fitness Plan

Dear Dr. Jock:

I've tried, I've tried, I've tried 4 different times to get started on an exercise program . . . and 4 times I've failed. Twice I pulled muscles and last time I got so bored with doing my daily dozen every day I just couldn't take it anymore. I've gained 14 pounds, I'm 44 years old, 5'4", 146 pounds, and I know I'm running out of time. Can you help?

T.S., Dallas, Texas

Dear Dr. Jock:

I'm a lawyer, 37, 6'1", 205, I smoke, I drink, and I'm in the worst physical shape of my life. Other than that, my life is going extremely well. My law associate died of a heart attack last month. We looked so much alike, people used to think we were brothers. I want to get myself into condition, but I don't know where to start. What kind of exercise would be good for me? How often should I do it? How long? If I start tomorrow when will I begin to see results?

A.D., Austin, Texas

Dear Dr. Jock:

I started to run a few weeks ago and I hated it. From beginning to end, the whole thing made me sick. My wife said she read somewhere that you can get just as fit from fast walking as you can from running. Is this possible? I'm much happier walking fast but if it's not going to help me get back into shape (I'm 30 pounds overweight and can't do 3 chin-ups), why bother? What do you say?

S.S., Gainesville, Florida

Lucy and Robin started an exercise program the same day. They remember it was a Monday—diets and exercise programs *always* start on a Monday, don't they?—and they took a vow on the last frozen Snickers bar in the house that this time, *this time,* they were serious.

They were going to forget all past efforts at getting started, forget about last year's slimnastics class, and the tennis lessons at the club two years ago, and the belly-dancing sessions at the Y, and they were especially going to forget how sick they got last spring when they tried to run to the 7-11 three blocks away without stopping.

Lucy went at it like a house afire. She'd been a cheerleader in high school and she dug out her old flare skirt from the 12th grade and hung it in her closet to remind her what a size 6 looks like. She bought a jogging suit, quickly skimmed a running book, borrowed her son's stopwatch and the first day out she clocked herself at a remarkable 8-minute half mile. It was also remarkable that she made it back to the house alive. At the age of 34, Lucy had the body of a 54-year-old woman. In her eagerness finally to get herself back in shape, she overdid it—as so many people do when they first decide to exercise.

Lucy spent that first week pushing and pulling herself into total exhaustion. By Sunday night she felt as though every muscle in her body had been turned inside out. On Monday, when Lucy managed to drag herself out of bed for what was to be her eighth straight day of exercise, she never made it past her bowl of Wheaties. She felt awful. Why punish herself, she thought? Who needs it? Her body was weak and her spirit totally unwilling to keep going. So she stopped. Like most people who begin regular exercise programs with the best of intentions, Lucy became a fitness fad dropout. She felt fat and a failure and she avoided seeing her friend Robin for weeks.

Meanwhile, Robin had taken a different approach to getting fit. It was several weeks before she worked up to her first mile of running, but she refused to worry. She knew if she stuck with it long enough the first mile mark would come, followed by the 2nd, then 5 and 8 or 10 if she wanted. The Boston Marathon is what she really wanted. But all she desired at the beginning was to keep going. She hurt too, but she didn't panic. She knew if she kept at it and kept stretching out her tight, tender muscles, they would eventually respond. Keep going, she told herself, that's the trick. She wasn't so sure she'd like running, so she signed up for racquetball lessons too, and alternated the two sports for 4 days a week. On Sundays she rested, and on Tuesday and Thursday too. On the days she did work out, she was careful not to drive herself to the point of exhaustion. She'd start out walking a block, running a block, walking a block and when she finally worked her way up to her first, full, 15-minute-mile of slow, continuous running, she was thrilled. So what if she was passed along the way by a blind runner and a housewife pushing a baby in a stroller? Robin didn't mind playing tortoise to the hares of the world as long as she could sustain herself for 30 minutes of exercise, not a moment less and sometimes more.

Some days, the 30 minutes seemed like an eternity and the only pleasure came from stopping. But some days—and this happened more and more as Robin kept at it—her 30 minute run flew by. On those days, her mind was clear and her breathing was steady, and she could soak up the simple pleasure of running while she thought out problems or simply looked at pretty boats along the lakefront.

You can probably see where this story is going. After a few weeks of discipline, tempered with common sense and uncommon determination, Robin was well on the road to achieving fitness.

No fitness program works if you don't stick to it. The biggest problem is sticking with it long enough to realize the benefits. Once that happens, once your natural body wisdom is allowed to take over and you begin to notice that you're looking better and feeling better than you ever felt before, the chances of your giving in to sloth or dropping out are greatly reduced.

Lucy never had a chance. She was in too much of a hurry. She was so busy thinking about how thin she could get, about how fast she should run, about how much pain she could endure, she forgot to have any fun at all. And if your exercise plan isn't fun, you might as well throw in the towel and go back to Monday Night Football.

But how can exercise be fun? How can you make it enjoyable enough so that you will continue? Here is where we can help. If you don't understand what you're doing, and why you're doing it, and how to do it safely, the chances are you'll wind up with Lucy, back on the sidelines, flabby and frustrated and wondering what went wrong. A little knowledge of the basics will go a long way toward keeping you going . . . and going . . . and going, no matter your age, sex, weight or prior fitness record. You're never too old to begin and it's never too late to start, so long as you take the proper precautions and begin the right way.

This chapter won't dictate a precise program, nor will it guarantee instant fitness or double-your-money-back. We don't really believe in one-size-fits-all programs. We prefer the "Fish Gotta Swim, Birds Gotta Fly" approach, taking into account the fact that running isn't for everyone—that for some the answer is swimming, for others it may be bicycling, and so on. Our plan is to supply enough facts so that you can explore the options and compile a fitness regimen that is right *for you*.

One of the facts we present is that you can improve your fitness in a variety of ways, choosing your sport or activity from a wide range of possibilities. Naturally, it has to be sufficiently vigorous to fit the minimum requirements for cardiovascular fitness, and in the chart on page 26 we've indicated which sports are your best bets for this. Later on in the book, we'll go into some of the more popular sports in greater detail (running, cycling, swimming, skiing, baseball, golf, racquet sports), and indicate how you can play it better, play it safer and enjoy it more.

While we won't dictate which sport you choose, we will help you develop an approach to any recreational sport, an attitude about fitness and exercise designed to keep you interested and keep you going. Keep going, that's the key to success. We can help you avoid quitting, by alleviating some of the pain and the guilt and the groveling for accomplishment that can kill the pleasure and make enjoyment nearly impossible. But first, a few words about fitness in general, so we'll all know what we're talking about.

WHAT IS FITNESS, ANYWAY?

There are many kinds of fitness. There is physical fitness, mental fitness, cardiovascular fitness, muscular fitness and more. Being fit involves all of these, but most important of all, it involves coping with all the stresses and messes of everyday life. Being fit involves more than just not being sick. We all know a lot of people who aren't wheezing or sneezing with some obvious illness, but who aren't in condition either. Good health can cover up their lack of fitness, but eventually gradual erosion catches up with them. Just because disease is absent doesn't mean you are enjoying your life to the fullest.

The AMA's Committee on Exercise and Physical Fitness defined fitness as "the general capacity to adapt to and respond favorably to physical effort." Naturally, being fit will also help you be the athlete you want to be: strong, confident, injury-free. If you're fit, not only will you do your sport better, you'll enjoy it more. And if you're fit, the saying goes, you may not increase the *quantity* of your years but you will assuredly improve the *quality*. And isn't that what life is all about, anyway?

Back to basics. For the purposes of talking about fitness in relation to exercise, we have to talk about a variety of factors: about strength, balance and flexibility, agility, power and endurance. This book spends a lot of time with flexibility and strength, but all of these go into making you fit, and all of these factors can be improved with work. The harder you work, the quicker you'll get fit . . . up to a point. And it's an important point for you to understand. You'll have to expend energy to get fit, but you don't have to—indeed, you should not—expend so much energy that you end up too hurt, or too exhausted, or too disappointed to go on. People drop out along the road to fitness usually because they are trying too hard, pushing too fast. Remember Lucy?

In sports medicine, we call it the overuse syndrome. And every year it's responsible for millions of pulled muscles, wrenched knees, torn Achilles and probably every case of tendinitis in town. So look for progress in your fitness program, but don't look for it too quickly, or too often. Don't be a slave to the stopwatch or forever interrupt your flow to take your pulse. It is important to check on your fitness level every so often—and this chapter will tell you how to do that—but try not to get so bogged down in cardiovascular details you miss the big, beautiful picture you are making of yourself.

MAXIMIZE YOUR ENERGY, MINIMIZE YOUR RISK

Hitting a tennis ball, schussing down a mountain, scrubbing floors, cycling through the countryside, planting petunias and running a 10-kilometer race have this in common—they all require you to exert energy. The more strenuous the activity, the more energy you expend. A leisurely stroll down the avenue may burn only 120–150 calories an hour, whereas steady walking at 5 or more mph can be a pretty good conditioner, using between 420 and 480 calories an hour, the energy equivalent of bicycling at 11 mph. The chart on page 26 gives the energy equivalent of your sport.

Muscles enable your body to expend energy to do work. There are 434 individual muscles in the human body, each with its own particular job to do, and all need energy to do it. You supply the energy in the form of glucose (blood sugar) and free fatty acids, which are broken down from the food you eat—primarily from the fats and carbohydrates; surprisingly little comes from the proteins. (More about this in Chapter 6.)

In order for your muscles to contract repeatedly—which is what muscles do best—you must make a constant supply of energy available to them. If you are able to supply a lot of energy at a fairly rapid rate, your muscles can do a lot of hard work. If your energy delivery system is a little sluggish and not operating anywhere near peak efficiency, your muscles will perform less well.

To get an energy delivery system working as near peak efficiency as possible, we have to look at how the cardiovascular system is working. That is the system that delivers oxygen throughout your body. Though you don't ordinarily think of your body as one great big oxygen machine, that's what it is. Shutting off the supply of oxygen will kill the motor almost as quickly as pulling the plug on a color TV kills the picture. For every 5 calories of energy you expend, according to the experts at the Human Performance Laboratory in Denver, you have to deliver about 1 liter of oxygen. If, for example, you're cross-country skiing up a gradual slope, your muscles will need about 15 calories of energy a minute—which is another way of saying that 3 liters of oxygen a minute must be transported to your muscles. If the supply is meeting the demand, and oxygen is being supplied at the rate necessary to produce the calories needed, the process called aerobic metabolism is taking place. Under such conditions, 67 percent of all the calories in the glucose available in your bloodstream are being converted to energy.

Sometimes, when special demands are made on the body, they may be greater than your ability to replenish the supply of oxygen. As a classic example, suppose a mugger is chasing you through the park. Your body, in the maximum exertion of trying to get away, is far outstripping your ability to deliver enough oxygen. Luckily, your muscle cells are equipped for such emergencies with a unique override system—supplying the necessary energy for getting away (we hope) *without oxygen,* by means of what is called anaerobic metabolism. Though it can be a lifesaver, anaerobic metabolism isn't nearly as efficient as aerobic metabolism. Without a supply of oxygen, only 3.5 percent of the calories in the available glucose are converted to energy. And though your body can do strenuous work in the absence of oxygen—sprinters run the 100-yard dash without taking a breath— the amount, and therefore the time, is limited. Two minutes is the absolute upper limit; often it is no more than one minute.

Anaerobic metabolism is useful in certain kinds of advanced athletic training, but we're mainly concerned in this book with the fundamentals of aerobic exercise. To do the kind of work that most recreational athletes are concerned with, oxygen has to be present. And that's what cardiovascular fitness is all about—training your body to furnish more oxygen, along with the other essential nutrients, over a longer period of time.

BOOSTING YOUR OXYGEN, STRENGTHENING YOUR HEART

Your body takes in oxygen through the respiratory passages and into the lungs. With training, the amount of air taken in with each breath can be increased. One way of doing this is by strengthening the respiratory muscles of the diaphragm and the muscles between the ribs. Many of us tend to be very shallow breathers, and this means that we are not using our lung capacity as efficiently as we could. There are now all sorts of disciplines—deep breathing exercises, yoga and body awareness programs—that focus on controlled abdominal breathing.

Once the good stuff, the oxygen, enters your lungs, it is exchanged for the bad stuff, the carbon dioxide, that collects in the alveoli, the tiny terminal air sacs inside the lungs. They turn dark and stop functioning properly when you smoke or inhale pollutants for too long. Breathing efficiently means taking into the blood as much oxygen as you can, and getting rid of as much CO_2 as you can. The rate of exchange depends on how fast the blood, with its supply of oxygen, passes *through* the lungs. And the major factor in the entire process of delivering oxygen throughout the tissues of the body is the efficiency of the cardiac muscle that does the pumping—in other words, your heart.

If that pump is weak, you're going to have problems. With each beat or contraction, the heart expels a certain amount of blood. This amount is called the stroke volume, and it depends on the rate and force of the contraction: the number of beats, the force of each beat. Like any other muscle in the body, the cardiac pump responds to proper exercise. If you work to strengthen it, you can increase the force of each contraction. Greater force means greater efficiency, and the more efficient your heart is, the better off you are.

How do you measure that efficiency? It's simple. The output of the heart per minute is determined by the stroke volume times the number of beats per minute. People who are fit have slower pulses when they are at rest because their hearts have to beat less often to furnish all the blood, oxygen and nutrients they need. In short, their hearts are more efficient. That's one of the things fitness does for you. The normal resting heart rate is about 72 beats per minute, but in a conditioned athlete it may be as low as 40. (Does getting more work out of fewer beats mean he'll live longer? We're not sure, but we're willing to bet he'll live *better*.)

Cardiac output, the amount of blood your heart pumps per minute, can increase up to 9 times its resting value as a result of exercise. Since the maximum heart rate is about 200 beats per minute in an adult (or about 3 times the normal resting rate), the remainder of the cardiac output must come from an increased stroke volume. A person who is physically fit has the strength in his or her heart muscle to increase the stroke volume, and since the resting pulse is slower, the rate can be increased to 4 or 5 times the normal rate and still not risk going over the safely attainable maximum rate. All of which adds up to what we already know about fit people: they can do more work over a longer period of time.

Fitness—in this instance, the development of endurance—very likely causes some changes at the muscular level too, so that the oxygen and nutrients that are being delivered more efficiently can also be utilized more efficiently. Though this is a controversial question (about which expert studies are now being made), we can assume that the ability of the muscle cell to bind and utilize the available oxygen increases substantially with increased fitness. Art Dickinson and Ken Sparks of the Human Performance Laboratory at the University of Denver have reported that, in fit people, "the energy-producing constituents of the muscle cells, the mitochondria, and the enzymes that biochemically reduce fats and carbohydrates to useful energy, may double in number or activity." They also report that capillaries, where oxygen is delivered to the cell and carbon dioxide is picked up, increase greatly and make the total system all the more efficient. It's no wonder, with all these changes occurring up and down the line and

VALUE OF VARIOUS EXERCISES

	Approx. cal. used per hour	Fitness benefits	Fitness deficits
Running 10 mph	900	Excellent conditioner	Many overuse injuries
Jogging 5 mph	500	Good conditioner	Can be tedious, some stress
Walking 2½ mph	200	Good for older people	Must be done for extended periods
Swimming ¼ mph	300	Good for people with bad backs; excellent conditioner	Wet hair
Cycling 13 mph	660	Excellent conditioner	Sore bottom; cars and dogs
Cycling 6 mph	275	Good conditioner	Duration of runs too short
Skiing downhill	550	Promotes skill	
Skiing cross-country	800	Excellent conditioner	Need snow
Tennis—singles	400	Good conditioner if done often enough	Tennis elbow
Tennis—doubles	350	Good social mixer	Not hard enough to improve fitness
Squash, racquetball, handball	600	Very good conditioner if done often enough	Court time can be expensive; stop/start injuries, too
Golf—walking	350	Improves fitness if done frequently enough Gets you outdoors	Clubs get heavy
Golf—power cart	200		$18/round
Bat and ball	250	Team play	Not sufficient to increase your fitness

throughout the entire body, that fitness has the effect it does. We feel different because we are different. We've changed ourselves in the most basic way.

FITNESS DEPENDS ON INTENSITY, DURATION, FREQUENCY

To achieve cardiovascular fitness, you have to strive for what doctors call a training effect. In other words, you have to make your heart work harder than it normally does, through demanding more of your body than it is used to. That's called *intensity*. Then you have to sustain that demand for a certain length of time—so you need *duration*. Then you have to repeat that demand on a certain schedule—and that means *frequency*.

INTENSITY—PUSH, BUT DON'T PUNISH

Intensity is the most flexible and, to some degree, the least important factor in fitness. You don't have to make a 100 percent effort to achieve a training effect. To do that would be self-defeating; you'd wear yourself out before you got anywhere. You can benefit from a training effect by working at from 60 to 85 percent of the maximum effort. Most serious competing athletes train at from 80 to 85 percent of their maximum; but that would be an unrealistically high goal if you're just starting out. You may want to reach that goal one day—and you can—but to get there, make sure that you build up to it gradually.

How do you determine your maximal heart rate? One easy, safe way is to go and see a health professional. We realize most people are not going to do this, nor is it necessary for everyone, but if you are over forty and have been sedentary all your life, or if you are plagued by fears that once you start running you'll drop dead on the track, then you probably ought to begin your program with a stress cardiogram. This is an EKG taken while you are running on a treadmill. An ordinary EKG, taken at rest, won't answer the question of how your heart will respond under stress; you have to stress it first and have a doctor nearby to evaluate the results.

If you want, and can afford, to go further in getting a professional evaluation, you might consider having a comprehensive fitness examination, which is becoming more and more popular across the country. In Chicago, for instance, Dick Hoover, who is physical therapist and trainer to the Sting soccer team, started a service called Fitness Analysis, for evaluating overall fitness and prescribing an individualized program to get people back into shape. Hoover and the staff determine your maximum capacity for exertion with a treadmill test for cardiovascular and respiratory functions. They also assess your flexibility and come up with a complete picture of your muscular strength. Body measurements are taken to determine the actual percentage of fat in your body—a more reliable indicator of overweight than the little charts you find in a 69-cent calorie counter booklet. When they're done, you come away with an exercise prescription— which will turn out to be absolutely worthless unless you decide to put in the time and effort to make it work.

If you're in reasonably good health and you don't feel up to the expense and bother of a stress test or a comprehensive fitness analysis, you can determine your own maximum heart rate, and come up with your own exercise prescription. First, subtract your age from the number 220. The figure you get is your maximal heart rate. To produce a training effect, you should swim or run or bicycle or otherwise work long enough and hard enough to push your pulse to between 60 and 85 percent of that figure, and then keep it there for at least 15 minutes. We've already worked this out for you, and broken it down into 10-second times in the chart on page 00. See the caption for detailed instructions on how to use it.

If, for example, you're 45 years old, operating at 60 percent, max means your pulse is going along at 19 beats every 10 seconds; 85 percent of max means 25 beats every 10 seconds. Generally speaking, we say shoot for 75 percent of max; but this is a qualified recommendation, depending on your age, your condition and what you're trying to accomplish. If you're a 17-year-old basketball player trying to build up endurance for college tryouts, you might want to train at 85 percent, but if you're a flustered, flabby stockbroker who hasn't lifted anything heavier than the Yellow Pages in twenty-five years, you should be happy to hit 60 percent. The catch is, if you *are* that out-of-shape beginner, it's likely that the first few times you work out and take your pulse, you'll find it's racing like mad, possibly registering more than 25 beats in 10 seconds, or higher than 85 percent. Instead of patting yourself on the back, you should slow down. Since you're working at an unrealistically intense pace, chances are that you won't be able to sustain it for the required 15 minutes. If you persist in pushing too hard, and work at too intense a level, you are very likely going to drop out. Remember Lucy?

When you're aware of your own body, you won't really need to check your pulse against the sweep hand on your watch to know how hard you're working. Your body will tell you when it's time to slack off. One good way to avoid pushing yourself too hard is to make sure that you can carry on a fairly normal conversation while you work out. This is an especially important test for runners—even if it means talking to yourself, or singing, or reciting as much as you can remember of the Gettysburg Address. If your breathing is so out of control that you can't speak, you are probably pushing yourself too hard. (You will want to push that hard if anaerobic training is what you're after, but it must be worked up to gradually.) If you're regularly wheezing and gasping for air as you run, you are probably going too fast. Being able to control your breathing is not simply one of the benefits of getting fit; it's something you should focus on all along the way.

Remember, the intensity of your exercise (as measured by your pulse rate) is only one factor in achieving fitness. Duration and frequency—how long you exercise, and how often—are, as we've said, much more important to the success of your program. You're much better off working like Robin, at a slower pace for a longer period of time, than you are pushing yourself and your pulse so hard that you take all the fun away.

Working out should be fun, not all the time, and not a real knee-slapper of a good time, like a vintage Chaplin film, but it should have its moments of pleasure that are so sweet, so seductive, that they keep you coming back for more. You'll miss some of that if you push too hard. You'll run right over it and then you'll wonder what it is people see in running anyway, it's so painful and boring. Your plan for getting fit, playing sports, is only as boring and painful as you make it.

There is another reason for gearing yourself to a lower intensity program besides boosting your enjoyment. Your body will tolerate it better, and you'll injure yourself less. And while you're cutting down your risk of injury, you're not compromising your fitness in the least. That's the interesting part. Walking is certainly a lower intensity activity than running, yet researchers have found out that a 40-minute, 4-times-a-week walking program did as much to improve the fitness of a test group of middle-aged men as a 30-minute, 3-day-a-week, moderate jogging program. The walking was certainly less strenuous, but the difference was offset by increased duration and frequency of training. A smart recreational athlete is patient enough to slow down and go on a little longer.

DURATION: KEEP MOVING AT LEAST 30 MINUTES

So once you decide on the kind of exercise you want to do—running, swimming, cycling or whatever—you need to know not only how long you should keep at it, but also how frequently. As we've said, in order to achieve a training effect, you have to raise your pulse to at least 60 to 85 percent of maximum and keep it there for at least 15 minutes. Since you will need some time to work up to it, and also some time to cool down afterward, you should plan on exercising for at least 30 minutes at a time.

It's fine, and even desirable, to exercise for a longer period than that. But you should make a hard and fast rule that you're not going to quit before the half hour is up—even if that means you have to go from a run to a jog, or from a jog to a walk. The important thing is to keep moving, feel comfortable and stay with it. That's the reasoning behind long, slow-distance exercising (slower pace, longer duration), and the benefits are enormous. But to enjoy those benefits you have to get over the initial hump, which usually comes in the first 10 or 15 minutes of exercise, when every fiber of your being is telling you to stop.

Why 10 or 15 minutes? No one quite knows. Kris Berg, a professor at the University of Nebraska, says it's a fact "that most people have a time consciousness that governs their lives, and it may take 10 to 15 minutes to disassociate from a mental calendar and timetable." That sounds right to us. If you resist this initial urge to quit ("I have a headache today, I'd better not go swimming," or "It looks like rain, maybe I should run tomorrow morning instead," or "What am I doing out here, when I don't feel like cycling?"), your mind will eventually stop giving you trouble and you'll begin to notice that you're feeling a whole lot better than when you started. If you stick with it 45 minutes or more, or maybe a little less, you may sometimes get into another plane altogether—the high, the flow, the immediate pleasure that athletes experience as an extra bonus of keeping fit.

FREQUENCY: THREE TIMES A WEEK, OR EVERY OTHER DAY

If some vigorous exercise is good, isn't more necessarily better? Not really. According to the best research to date, you're best off exercising for cardiovascular fitness 3 times a week, or every other day. You can improve your heart-lung system by working out twice a week, but to do so you have to push yourself extremely hard, and most people would find exercising at that intensity impossible to continue. Besides, working out 3 times a week is much more likely to produce noticeable changes in body weight and contour—a smaller waist, a flatter stomach, slimmer legs.

The same research (reported by Dr. Michael Pollock, director of the Cardiac Rehabilitation Center for the Evaluation of Human Performance at the Wisconsin–Mount Sinai Medical Center in Milwaukee) concluded that training 5 days a week was too much. It's workable for some folks, but most of us have busy schedules, demanding businesses and families and other obligations. Finding time to work out 5 days a week is unrealistic, though certainly not unheard of. The benefits of exercising more than 5 days a week proved minimal.

Three days a week seems like a happy compromise. It's just enough to develop cardiovascular-respiratory fitness but it's not too much to commit yourself to. And for beginning runners, it's an especially good number to remember since the Pollock study showed that the injury rate related to the foot, ankle and knee joints increased dramatically when joggers trained more than 3 days per week. In one group of young men, the ones exercising 5 days a week had three times as many injuries as the ones holding themselves to 3. They concluded, and we wholeheartedly agree, that the body needs to rest in between workouts. If you push too hard, too fast, you set yourself up for injuries or failure or both. Even accomplished, experienced athletes who keep up their exercise regimens 5 days a week or more are sure to intersperse hard days with easy days; for example, they will alternate days running and sprinting with something less demanding on the legs, like swimming and bicycling. No one wants to be guilty of overtraining. It's exhausting and it's wasteful and sometimes you end up leaving your best effort on the practice track.

PUTTING IT ALL TOGETHER AND WRITING IT DOWN

To summarize briefly, your ideal fitness program should meet the following three requirements: (1) INTENSITY—your activity should be vigorous enough to push your pulse to between 60 and 85 percent of maximum and keep it there for about 15 minutes; (2) DURATION—you should plan on exercising at least 30 minutes, and longer if possible; (3) FREQUENCY—at the start, plan to work out 3 days a week. Every other day may be even better.

Once you've settled on your basic program, invest in a fresh, clean steno pad and write down what you're going to do, and when, and how often. If your aim is to lose weight or trim off inches or chase away the blues, record that too. Keep it loose and informal. Since you're the one it's addressed to, be honest with yourself. Every time you work out, make a note of it, even if it's no more than the date and a series of expletives.

Some days you'll feel like writing nothing and some days you'll surprise yourself and the words and feelings will flow like crazy. Don't push it, just keep going. By keeping track, you'll help yourself stay on track. You do this, the behavior mod experts say, by increasing your awareness of the whole process. The process is much more important than the progress. If you stick to it, you'll make progress, there's no question of that. But if you give up on the process of getting fit, if you can't find some enjoyment every time you work out, if you can't appreciate what you're going through while you are going through it, you'll probably stop. Keep your journal going, and you'll keep going too.

OUR SEPARATE AND EQUAL CLAUSE

Fitness is an equal opportunity enterprise. Though there are some differences between men and women (for instance, women tend to have more body fat, less arm strength), none of them are obstacles to developing fitness. This goes for the older athletes, too. Some of the happiest, best letters we get are from men and women who discovered fitness late in life. They took their time, and many did it with a doctor standing nearby just in case. But by sticking to the concept of slower pace and longer distance and letting up a bit on the intensity of the workout, large numbers of people 65 and older are discovering that growing older may not be reversible, but it's a heckuva lot more fun if you keep yourself active, fit and flexible.

FOUR STEPS TO CHECKING YOUR FITNESS

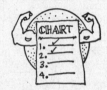

To achieve a training effect, you must push your pulse to between 60 and 85 percent of your maximal heart rate, and keep it there at least 15 minutes.

1. Exercise 10 minutes and count your pulse for 10 seconds.
2. Find your age and maximal heart rate and see how hard you're working.
3. Keep going at least 30 minutes. Slow down, or speed up, as necessary.
4. Remember: checking the intensity of your exercise is important, but don't get bogged down with numbers.

Age	Maximal heart rate	60% (10 sec)	65% (10 sec)	70% (10 sec)	75% (10 sec)	80% (10 sec)	85% (10 sec)
20	200	20	22	23	25	27	28
21	199	=	=	=	=	=	=
22	198	=	=	=	=	26	=
23	197	=	=	=	=	=	=
24	196	=	=	=	24	=	27
25	195	=	=	=	=	=	=
26	194	=	=	=	=	=	=
27	193	=	=	=	=	=	=
28	192	=	21	22	=	25	=
29	191	=	=	=	=	=	=
30	190	19	=	=	=	=	=
31	189	=	=	=	=	=	=
32	188	=	=	=	=	=	=
33	187	=	=	=	23	=	26
34	186	=	=	=	=	=	=
35	185	=	20	=	=	=	=
36	184	=	=	21	=	=	=
37	183	=	=	=	=	24	=
38	182	=	=	=	=	=	=
39	181	=	=	=	=	=	=
40	180	18	=	=	=	=	=
41	179	=	=	=	22	=	25
42	178	=	=	=	=	=	=
43	177	=	=	=	=	=	=
44	176	=	19	=	=	23	=
45	175	=	=	20	=	=	=

Age	Maximal heart rate	60% (10 sec)	65% (10 sec)	70% (10 sec)	75% (10 sec)	80% (10 sec)	85% (10 sec)
46	174	"	"	"	"	"	"
47	173	"	"	"	"	"	24
48	172	"	"	"	21	"	"
49	171	"	"	"	"	"	"
50	170	17	"	"	"	"	"
51	169	"	"	"	"	"	"
52	168	"	"	"	"	22	"
53	167	"	"	19	"	"	"
54	166	"	18	"	"	"	"
55	165	"	"	"	"	"	23
56	164	"	"	"	"	"	"
57	163	"	"	"	"	"	"
58	162	"	"	"	"	"	"
59	161	"	"	"	20	21	"
60	160	16	"	"	"	"	"
61	159	"	"	18	"	"	"
62	158	"	"	"	"	"	"
63	157	"	"	"	"	"	"
64	156	"	"	"	"	"	"
65	155	"	"	"	"	"	22
66	154	"	"	"	"	"	"
67	153	"	"	"	"	"	"
68	152	"	"	"	"	"	"
69	151	"	"	"	"	"	"
70	150	"	"	"	"	"	"

10 SIMPLE STEPS TOWARD YOUR OWN FITNESS PROGRAM

1. Buy a clean, fresh notebook and title it something elegant like *My Fitness Journal.* You can write on the backs of old shirt cardboard but keeping track of your progress in a separate notebook makes everything so much more official.

2. Check out the chart on page 26 and decide what activity or combination of activities you're going to do to make yourself fit. (If you choose golf or bowling, you might as well get your money back on the notebook.) Running, swimming, cycling, fast walking, long distance skiing are traditionally best fitness sports.

3. Whatever you choose, plan to do it at least 3 times every week, at least 30 minutes each session. Work hard enough to have a training effect but not so hard that it's not fun. Don't do it every day or you'll burn yourself out. Give your body a chance to rest in between. Keep it happy; it'll keep you happy.

4. Write down the whole plan in the little notebook in as much detail as you want. Then follow the instructions for Keeping a Journal on page 31.

5. Take a vow, make a pledge, say a solemn oath that you will warm up religiously for at least 10 minutes before each exercise session. Every day is better but we'll take what we can get. The chart on pages 104–105 tells you about warm-ups.

6. Immediately follow that sacred promise with another, that you will take 5 to 10 minutes to cool down after you exercise. You will not stop dead and quit. If you do, you may feel sore the next day.

7. Every once in a while check your pulse to see how your fitness is improving but don't make a big deal out of it. Don't let your competitive instincts run your life.

8. Learn to listen to your body. It will tell you when you're overdoing it.

9. Strengthening exercises will help you perform better and prevent injuries. The chart on pages 152–153 will help you choose the ones that are most helpful.

10. Make your exercise program fun. If you don't, you'll be a drop-out. If you're a drop-out, please return to step 1.

4. Sports Injuries:

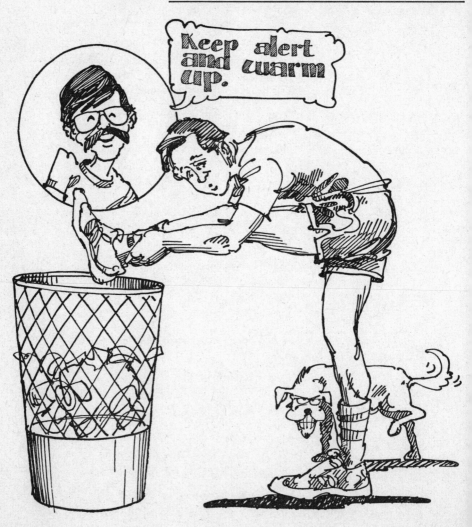

Prevention and Care

Dear Dr. Jock:

I did something bad to my knee (I think) when I was running. Normally, I can run about 8 to 10 miles a day, 5 or 6 times a week, but my knee hurts so much lately I've had to cut back. I went to my family doctor and he says I should stop running altogether. Says there's nothing I can do but rest and hope the pain goes away. Says running is for horses and for youngsters and then, after I told him how much I hated golf, he said he hated runners and was sick to death of their problems. I live in a little town and don't know what to do next. Are there any exercises I can do on my own that might help?

M.M., Yakima, Washington

Dear Dr. Jock:

What's in a bruise? Is there a medicine I can take to make one go away? Is it dangerous? Why is it different colors? My mom told me drinking a lot of milk will help it go away faster. Is that true?

S.G., Knoxville, Tennessee

Dear Dr. Jock:

I'm an avid tennis player, 5'9", good health, 43 years old, 163 pounds. Last year, I came down with a bad case of tendinitis. I went to my doctor and he told me to lay off tennis until it felt better. I stopped for a week or so then started again, and again the pain was intense. I went back and he gave me some pills to take. They made me sleepy and I still had pain when I played. I heard about another doctor who did acupuncture (it didn't help) and then I tried ultrasound therapy but my tendinitis still hung on. Now another doctor wants to give me cortisone shots. I've spent a fortune trying to get rid of it and I don't know what to do anymore. What do you advise? (Are cortisone shots supposed to be safe?)

L.P., Los Angeles, California

The body in motion is a wondrous array of moving parts—muscles, ligaments, joints, tendons and bones—and each part is vulnerable to physical stress and mental strain. Sports-medicine people tend to lump all sports-related injuries into two handy categories: those due to accidents and those due to overuse. Occasionally, though, there's an injury that falls through the cracks and makes a point all its own.

Take the case David had a while back involving Bobby, a 16-year-old athlete with a serious knee problem. Bobby, who was on the school football team, kept having to miss practice and games because of a painful, swollen left knee. He hadn't been in any accident, and he seemed to respond to a program of rest and strengthening exercises, but every time he'd go back to playing again, the same agonizing problem would recur. David was baffled; he'd done all the usual tests and X-rays and couldn't find a thing wrong.

Bobby's father had been a great ballplayer in college and was determined to have his son go to the same Ivy League school and play on the team. So he was absolutely beside himself, because the more determined he became, the more trouble Bobby had with his knee. Then, one day, David discovered the cause of the problem. Every time the boy's knee got red and swollen, it was because the poor kid was beating it with a hairbrush. Bobby didn't like football. He hated the thought of playing for his dad's old team. Rather than face the situation and tell his dad the truth, the kid chose to batter away at a perfectly healthy knee.

Parental pressure—or what kids perceive as parental pressure—is one of those hidden menaces when it comes to dealing with young athletes. The natural instinct of kids simply to have a good time can be easily subverted by an overbearing parent who can't stand to see his kid batting eighth in Little League, and by undertrained coaches, who still think that drinking water during football practice is for sissies.

You probably don't have to worry about pushy parents or overzealous coaches. You're on your own. The treatment you accept from your doctor is your responsibility. This chapter will help you cope.

AWARENESS PREVENTS ACCIDENTS; WARM-UPS PREVENT INJURIES

Most often, accidents happen because you've done something stupid. You're tense, you're not concentrating, you haven't taken the time to learn the sport properly or you've failed to check out the playing field. If you ride your bicycle in Chicago's rush hour traffic while your mind is shuffling off to Buffalo, you are asking for an accident. So the advice is be aware and stay alert. Check your equipment before you use it. Scan the playing field and remove loose tennis balls, broken glass or any other obstacle to your success and safety. It costs you only a minute and it could save all the ligaments in your ankle.

Probably the single most impressive statistic in sports medicine is that 80 percent of all injuries related to recreational sports are preventable. That's because 80 percent of those injuries are caused by lack of flexibility or overuse, and both of these are things you can learn to avoid. The best way to do that is to warm up your body, loosen up your muscles and joints before and after you work out. *This is probably the single most important piece of advice we can give you.*

STRETCH THOSE MUSCLES

Muscles are torn or pulled because they're so tight and inflexible that they give way when sudden force is applied to them. Naturally, active sports involve a lot of sudden force. If the muscle you're using is loose enough to stretch, it won't tear. Notice that we didn't say *strong* enough. Strong muscles are no substitute for flexible muscles. You need both for maximum protection against injury and for maximum enjoyment of your sport. Weight lifters who don't keep flexible can easily become muscle-bound; though they may look like perfect specimens, in fact they will be much more prone to injury in a 5-mile run than your neighbor down the block who spends a good half hour a day stretching out before he begins. You don't have to spend 30 minutes a day warming up to protect yourself, but if you spend any less than 10, you'll only be cheating yourself.

You can stretch and flex at any time of day, but loosening up just before you actually begin your sport is a must. Some athletes like to divide their warm-up routine, doing 10 minutes before and then 10 minutes more afterward, when they're feeling loose, and when the stretching helps cool them down. When you warm up isn't nearly as important as *how* you do it, and how often. Consistency is the key. Your body didn't get tight in a day; don't expect to loosen it up in a few minutes. Flexibility takes work, but it is your first and most important line of defense against injuries.

There are two types of stretching exercise—the static stretch and the ballistic stretch. Ballistic stretching is the bouncy kind and it is not recommended. It goes along with the masochistic, macho-istic philosophy of fitness that it's only good for you if it hurts—a philosophy that isn't recommended here either. In some European nations the experts are still big on ballistic stretching; but our best experts prefer a gentler and less violent process, which doesn't put nearly the force and strain on the fragile muscle fibers. If you attack your warm-up instead of embracing it, you can do yourself more harm than good. You are better off easing and exhaling your muscles into doing what you want them to do. When you stretch, string out the word s-t-r-e-t-c-h in your mind and let it float there for a while. Shift your focus to the muscle you are trying to warm up.

What does it feel like? Is it especially tight today? Take a few deep belly breaths and see if you can get it to relax. Don't force that issue either; the more you tell yourself to relax, the tougher it is to just let it naturally happen. Bring your mind into play because it'll help. Visualize your muscle as it stretches and feel all the tight tiny muscle fibers free up under the flow of blood. Once you feel the pull, hold it, relax, exhale and stretch a little farther. Repeat the exercise at least 5 times. There is an art to warming up properly and the sooner you learn it, and learn to enjoy it, the better off you'll be. We'll discuss which warm-ups are best for which sports in Chapter 7, and deal with various body parts, but for the time being, get busy and think of a way to make time for your warm-up ritual. Everyone can steal 10, even 20 minutes out of a day. You can stretch anywhere: in the car or the kitchen, in your office or on the phone. It's one of the basic principles of self-care and if you can't find time for it, you better ask yourself why.

TENDINITIS: THE OVERUSE SYNDROME

Overuse is a term you'll hear a lot in connection with sports-related injuries. A patient comes in with an aching knee after running 5 miles a day for 3 months. His warm-up routine consists of 3 minutes of jumping-jacks, a few toe-touches, some sit-ups and a beer. His knee never used to hurt before, but now it's killing him. "What's wrong, doc?" The same thing that's wrong with the tennis-mad stockbroker who took up the game at 34 and is trying to make up for lost time by playing 3 sets a day, 5 days a week. Both these players have a very common kind of sports-related injury called tendinitis. What causes it? You do. You are responsible for your own tendinitis because it means you have put your body through too much, too soon, without enough preparation.

Tendinitis comes from too little strength, too little flexibility and too much use. An arm that is normally used just to push a pen, steer a power-driven car or lift a slice of pizza is not in shape to hit tennis balls for two hours. You have to get it into shape, or you will suffer the consequences. If your arm isn't stretched and strengthened before you put stress on it, you will get microscopic tears in the muscle or tendon attachment. Those little injuries to the tendon may go completely unnoticed by you, at first, because your body will have healed itself before you even realize that damage was done. But as your body heals itself, what you're left with is scar tissue, which tears very easily. And when *it* gets torn, that's what really hurts. Indeed, that's the reason for the pain and swelling and distress of tendinitis. One important thing to remember always is that in time the problem will go away all by itself. The scar tissue will become healthy tendon tissue; and if you're faithful to your warm-ups, it won't happen again.

So the good news is that, almost certainly, you don't have to quit tennis because you've developed tennis elbow, and you needn't stop running just because your patellar tendon is acting up. You won't be making your condition any worse and continuing to play doesn't seem to slow down the process of healing—though you have to bear in mind that the process may take a very long time, sometimes even years. You don't need to keep running to a doctor during that time unless, of course, the situation gets worse instead of better. You can treat your own tendinitis very simply and safely, while the body heals itself.

HOW TO TREAT YOUR TENDINITIS

Generally speaking, all tendinitis is treated in the same way:

1. Before you begin to warm up and play, apply heat to the injured area for a few minutes. Relax and enjoy the soothing sensations. This can be done with a heating pad before you leave your house; better yet, go into the field house or club locker room and let hot (but not too hot) water run over the area. With a shoulder tendinitis this can get a little sloppy, so you may need to think about using a hot pack of some kind. Heat ointments and liniments may help a bit to warm the area, but they're more expensive and not nearly as good as ordinary tap water.

2. Stretch out the injured area, slowly and fully. Don't give in to its stiffness. Work on making it as loose and flexible as you can. Relax, exhale and work it a little farther.

3. Work out a program of strengthening exercises to be done at home. This is especially important in avoiding a reinjury. Chapter 8 will tell you which strengthening exercises to use.

4. After playing, get some ice on the painful area as soon as possible. Use an ice pack, or carry a coolerful of cubes and a plastic bag with you if you have to, but get it on as soon as you can. The miserable pain of tendinitis comes from swelling afterward, so the sooner you can get ice onto it and prevent the swelling, the farther you can go toward dealing with the pain. You can use the ice as necessary, 3 or 4 times a day, 15 or 20 minutes at a time. If the pain becomes too intense, you probably ought to see a doctor.

Whatever you do, don't come home with a case of tendinitis and run for the heating pad. It will not help you and it probably will make matters worse. If your mother insists on doing something to make you more comfortable, let her fix a pot of chicken soup.

LISTEN TO YOUR BODY

What happens in tendinitis and other overuse syndromes (described in Chapter 16, "Hot Spots—The Body Owner's Manual") needn't happen to you, so long as you are diligent about flexibility and strengthening exercises (see Chapters 7 and 8), and are careful not to push yourself too hard. How hard is too hard? It is a a good question, but you won't find the answer in any book or formula or scientifically tested program. You'll have to find the answer in your own reservoir of body wisdom. If you're like most people, it's largely untapped. We're taught to listen to Bach, and to car engines and birdcalls, but when it comes to listening to our own bodies, we're still pretty naive. Doctors help keep us that way by agreeing to listen to our bodies for us. Caring for yourself, though, means listening to your own body. Doing that is called body awareness, and there's nothing mystical or magical about it. It's a learnable skill, based on common sense plus the realization that the body is continually sending us signals, some of which we can readily interpret (such as pulse, heartbeat and respiration), along with others that we may have more trouble dealing with (such as pain, anxiety or tension). We have to learn to listen to those signals, to understand when the body is really exhausted, so that it would be dangerous to push on, and when it is simply acting leaden and lazy.

Increased body awareness and all the benefits that come with it—less stress, better performance, greater concentration, fewer injuries—constitute a whole subject in themselves. You'll find more about it in Chapter 5.

CAN I CONTINUE PLAYING?

Let's assume that in spite of regular warm-ups and your best efforts at listening to body wisdom, you do suffer a sports injury. As an active, sports-minded person, the first question you're going to ask yourself—and then your doctor—is whether you can continue to play or not. How do you know whether to keep going or to stop so as not to make matters worse?

This is where sports medicine and traditional medicine sometimes come to a parting of the ways. If you're a runner with a sore leg, or if you're a tennis player with a throbbing, painful elbow, and you go see your friendly regular internist, he may tell you to stop everything until the pain goes away. It's a safe call for the doctor; but having to give up a regular program of running, or racquetball, or swimming, or cycling, may be more painful than the injury that brought you to the doctor in the first place. Sports-medicine experts are keenly tuned into the extreme frustration that prescribed inactivity can bring, and they are geared toward keeping their patients going. If the injury is self-limiting—that is, if it is a tendinitis or some other condition that will eventually heal and that won't get worse if you play in the meantime—you should not be discouraged from getting back to your game. Indeed, you should be encouraged to stay as active as you can, to do something to keep yourself fit while you're recovering. If your knee hurts so badly you can't run on it until it heals, a sports-minded doctor will probably turn you on to swimming, or possibly cycling.

How can you find a sports-medicine expert in your community? There are at least three professional organizations you can write to for advice: the American College of Sports Medicine (1440 Monroe Street, Madison, Wisconsin 53706), the American Orthopedic Society for Sports Medicine (430 North Michigan Avenue, Chicago, Illinois 60611) and the American Academy of Podiatric Sports Medicine (c/o Dr. Steven Subotnick, 19682 Hesperian Boulevard, Haywood, California 94541). Sports medicine is a rapidly developing specialty that cuts across dozens of different professions; so you may get some leads by checking with local hospitals, medical schools, holistic health centers, wellness clinics, trainers, coaches, physical educators, and high school, college and professional athletes. Finding the right doctor for you may be tricky and time-consuming, but it could mean the difference between keeping going and having to stop.

SOME INJURIES DEMAND REST

As a general rule, if your injury is the result of a sudden incident—a fall or a collision—you'll probably have to stop playing altogether and let it heal. You can't run off an ankle sprain. When a ligament is torn, it needs time to heal or the tear may get worse. The first principle of healing is rest. Toughing it out, grinning and bearing it, may make you a martyr with your team coach and a hero to your wife, but it may aggravate the injury and delay healing. In cases of gross abuse—about which we're beginning to hear protests from some smart professional team players—to go on running, playing or hitting may leave you crippled for life. Dick Butkus was heralded as one of the greatest Bears of all time; but now, years after the cheering has stopped, he is left with pain, a limp and a lot of bitterness about the big business of pro sports. His bread and butter involved toughing it out too hard, too long, but it was his job and he did it brilliantly. Your bread and butter is not dependent on your sports performance, so there's absolutely no excuse for you to risk a lifelong disability by returning to your sport before you have full functional recovery.

Your aches and pains, however, won't usually come from a sudden injury on the playing field. They'll be the more insidious problems, involing sore tendons and crippled muscles that are the gradual result of neglect and improper conditioning.

KNOWING WHEN YOU'RE BADLY HURT

Common sense will tell you when you are badly hurt. If, for instance, you are speeding downhill on your brand new fiberglass skis, hit a mogul, fly through the air totally out of control, skin a tree, bounce off a boulder, land in a heap, hear a loud crack and see your leg casually draped across your shoulders, it doesn't take a diagnostic genius to tell you you're in trouble. The problem in self-diagnosis comes with the more minor injuries. Is this sharp knee pain one that will go away, or is it one that is leading up to a major hurt and needs to be looked at? The best time to begin your evaluation is (1) *after* you've stopped crying, and (2) *before* a lot of swelling and reactive pain set in. The reason that sports teams like to have their doctors right on the scene at games is so they will have seen the injury happen, and can check the wounded player just after, when the first waves of pain subside and something called tissue shock sets in.

So you're injured—what do you do? First of all, don't panic, and don't abandon your senses. Settle yourself with a few deep breaths and think for a minute. Did you hear a loud snap or crack when you went down? Did you feel something tear? Do a body check. Does everything appear to be lined up and in place? Is your body giving you signals that you skied one run too many or played one set too long and that now you're in trouble? Are you feeling numb, nauseated, dizzy or dopey? If your body tells you to stay put until the stretcher comes, don't fight it. If you're feeling shaken up but basically okay, continue taking inventory. Wiggle your toes. Your fingers. Are they okay? Try to move the part that hurts. Can you move it in every direction without pain? Does it feel stable—all in one piece? If it's your leg, can you stand on it? Good. Can you walk on it? Fine. Are you able to run? Are you then able to start and stop, change directions, run backward? Can you perform all the moves your sport requires? If you can, then whatever you did to yourself wasn't so bad, and you can shake off the dirt and go back to playing.

If you can't do all the things we've mentioned, stop at the place where pain interferes. If you can't move it through an entire range of motion, if it doesn't feel stable, if you can't stand or walk on it, you need a doctor. Do yourself a big favor and get an X-ray done as fast as the nearest emergency room can accommodate you. The best time for an examination is early, before it swells. And don't expect the X-ray to give all the answers. The standard emergency-room X-ray can only tell whether or not you have a fracture. It can't reveal torn cartilage or a spasm.

If you do find yourself in an emergency-room situation, be alert, ask questions and, without making yourself too obnoxious make sure that the person who sees you gives you ample time and attention. You should be checked for sensation in the injured area, presence of a pulse, range of motion and stability of the joint. If the area is completely numb and missing a pulse, the situation is serious, requiring immediate care. If the joint is unstable, you can expect a cast or even an operation.

If you see a doctor, whether you're fresh off the basketball court with a crushed ankle, or you're there because a lame leg is interfering with your tennis game, make sure your doctor sees you and your injury in toto, not just as an isolated sore spot. Every part of your anatomy is interdependent with the other parts. If your doctor tries to examine your sore knee with your jeans rolled up and your shoes and socks still on, forget him. You may get symptomatic relief from him, but you're not likely to find the real cause of the problem. Both legs have to be examined thoroughly to make a real diagnosis; and even then, the problem may really be down in your shoes, because your arches have fallen, leaving your knees to take all the stress.

A doctor who is attuned to runners' problems may immediately think of an orthotic device to keep you going. Another doctor may tell you there is nothing to be done except to rest, pray and pay your bills on time. So be careful, and stay involved. Going to a doctor about your sports injury doesn't automatically relieve you of all responsibility. The more involved and cooperative you are, the better off you'll both be. Don't be afraid to ask questions, and insist on answers that are clear to you. If your doctor mumbles something about a Watson-Jones procedure, a torn this or sprained that, find out what he's talking about. Ask what he's doing for you, and insist on knowing what you can do for yourself. Can you play on the injury? What exercises can you do to bring about a speedier return to full function? How long will healing take? Sure, doctors are busy and they don't always take the time they should to explain things, but you have a right to some answers. You *also* have a responsibility to listen carefully and remember what your doctor says. Doctors' phone lines are filled every day with panicky patients calling up to ask questions that have already been answered, two or three times. It's one thing to be curious and quite another to make yourself obnoxious.

FIRST STEPS IN TREATING AN INJURY

Whether you go to a doctor or not, the initial treatment for an injury is the same.

Swelling occurs with every injury. Sometimes you can see it—as when a twisted ankle blows up to the size of your calf—and sometimes you can't—as in the swelling that goes with an Achilles tendinitis. What happens when you get swelling is that blood vessels are torn, and the blood leaks into the tissues. This usually doesn't occur instantly, upon impact, but develops gradually over a few hours. A lot of swelling within an hour after getting hurt is usually a sign of a serious injury.

Swelling itself is painful—which means that to ease the pain after any sort of sports injury you should do something to reduce the swelling. Grandma used to say, plenty of hot water and Epsom salts. Well, Grandma was wrong. *Heat increases swelling.* The initial treatment for just about any injury is the same: I-C-E: Ice, Compression and Elevation.

STEP ONE: ICE

Ice in a cold pack or a plastic bag does a number of helpful things. It eases pain by slowing down nerve conduction. It helps prevent muscle spasm. And it reduces the bleeding that is the cause of swelling. How long should you use it? That's a good question, though still a matter of some debate. We say you should use ice at least 48 hours after an injury—72 is probably even better—15 or 20 minutes at a time, at least 4 times a day. As long as there is any significant swelling, don't use a heating pad or soak in a hot tub, whatever your friends may advise. Heat can be useful for regaining motion in a joint after the swelling has disappeared. There are some therapists and trainers, though, who don't recommend heat at all. If you can't make up your mind what to do, stick with the ice.

STEP TWO: COMPRESSION

The next step in self-care after an injury is compression, which mechanically restricts the swelling. You get compression by wrapping the injured part in an elastic bandage. Be sure to use the proper size: a 2- or 3-inch bandage for the hand or wrist, a 3- or 4-inch bandage for the elbow or ankle, and a 6-inch bandage for the knee or thigh. Don't use a 4-inch bandage for the knee. It is too small to do much good, and since people tend to put it on too tightly, it may actually do harm.

No matter what you do, you'll get some swelling. So when you put on an elastic bandage, you should roll rather than stretch it on. Rolling it allows the bandage to stretch without becoming too tight. A bandage that is too tight will cause increased pain; or it may cause some numbness and restrict circulation. See the illustration on p. 47 for instructions on wrapping injured parts. There are many acceptable ways of doing this. Find the one that suits you best, and that gives you maximum support with the least amount of discomfort. You can tell if it's wrapped too tight by testing the color of your finger and toenail beds. Normally they are pink, and if you squeeze them they turn white. When you let the pressure off they should become pink again in a second or two. If they don't, the bandage is too tight. Loosen it and try again. Continue to use the bandage until the swelling has pretty much gone away and you don't feel the need for support. You'll know when that is.

STEP THREE: ELEVATION

This keeps the injured part above the level of the heart and helps drain blood and tissue fluid from the extremity. Normally, the heart pumps blood out to the arms and legs. Muscle action pumps it back to the heart. If you've hurt a muscle and can't use it normally, the blood-return muscle pump doesn't work as well. You can help it, and help yourself, by elevating it for passive drainage.

After you put on that elastic bandage, you'll get some swelling below it, usually in the fingers or the toes. It can't be helped—the bandage combined with the injury hampers the return circulation—and it's nothing to worry about. A great deal of swelling, however, means your bandage is too tight.

BRUISES AFTER AN INJURY

The other thing you can expect to see after a sports injury is black-and-blue discoloration. Don't waste your porterhouse on a bruise; it will go away eventually. With every injury you get some internal bleeding, no matter whether it's a bruise, a sprain, a strain or

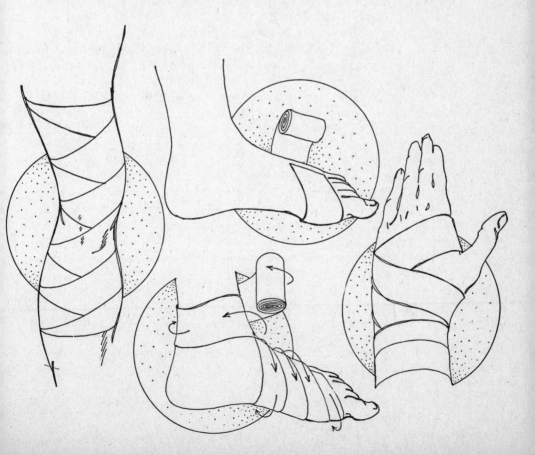

a fracture. And when there is bleeding inside, it shows up black-and-blue outside. In an ankle sprain, this blood will travel all over the foot, through the tissue planes. It will spread to the toes and if you've been elevating the foot the way you should, gravity will make it spread up to the leg. Don't be alarmed—it's normal.

One more word about black-and-blue. It becomes green-and-yellow as time passes. As the body decomposes the blood pigments, the color changes. If you're playing squash and get smacked in the thigh with the ball, you may not see anything for a few days. The first thing you do see will probably be a yellowish-green discoloration. That's a few-days-old bruise, finally rising to the surface.

CUTS AND PUNCTURES

As you're sliding into second, a piece of glass comes out of hiding and slashes your leg. Or your bicycle tire blows, you fall and scrape your arm and face. Such things can happen to anyone. Taking care of most skin wounds is pretty straightforward. Ordinary cuts and scrapes should be cleaned and left alone. Puncture wounds, especially if they are deep, need medical attention. Who knows what might be down in the depths of the hole? Deep cuts and puncture wounds that won't stop bleeding may need stitches, and that means seeing a doctor, even though he won't be able to make a wound heal any faster.

If your wound doesn't appear serious, begin by washing away all the dirt and bacteria, since they interfere with healing. So do foreign bits such as glass or gravel. Plain warm water will wash all that away, and a mild soap will help break down the fat on the skin and the wound surfaces so that the water can work even better. First-aid kits may be comforting to have around, but there is really no need to use any ointments or antiseptic solutions. If these solutions were strong enough to kill all the bacteria they would also be strong enough to damage the tissues, and damaged tissue heals more slowly than normal tissue. An ointment on the wound is just another foreign material. The best thing to do after washing off a wound is to let it hang out in the air to dry. It is good to let a scab form, so as to seal bacteria out and promote healing. Use a bandage only if the wound is going to be too much of a mess otherwise; bandages tend to keep the wounded area warm and moist, and that is the kind of place bacteria grow best in.

THE HEALING PROCESS

A lot of people are confused about healing. They think it's something done to them by doctors who have some secret about how to "cure" their weak, ailing bodies—generally with drugs, pills, ointments and assorted pharmaceuticals, all of them expensive. That certainly is the impression thrust upon us by million-dollar ad campaigns, but the truth is that drugs and doctors don't heal you, your body heals itself. Drugs and doctors and hospitals get all the credit (and a lot of cash, too), but as Dr. Ronald Glasser put it in his book on our natural defense system, *The Body Is the Hero:*

> There are a growing number of facts available that show plainly that we are as much a part of our own diseases as we are of our health, that we should be able to and indeed can help ourselves. The task of the physician today is what it has always been, to help the body do what it has learned to do so well on its own during its unending struggle for survival—to heal itself. It is the body, not medicine, that is the hero.

Doctors can be helpful, especially when it comes to the miracle of mechanical repair—total hip replacements, artificial heart valves, lifesaving coronary bypass operations, corneal transplants, etc. Some doctors are experimenting with small electrical currents to reduce normal bone healing time by 50 percent, and to speed up the mending of soft-tissue wounds too. But for the time being, the actual process of healing is done entirely by your body. The sooner you discover ways to help this process along—or, at least, stay out of its way while it's happening—the faster you'll be able to return to full-scale sports activity.

The healing process is a complicated chain of events involving inflammation, formation of new tissue, ingrowth of new blood vessels, skin growth, collagen ingrowth, enzyme activity and the central nervous system, to name just a few major links. If there's a weak link in that entire process making it less efficient, you can unconsciously slow the process down. If you're not dealing well with stress, for instance, or if your arteries are so clogged that your blood circulation is hampered, or if you're taking the wrong combination of drugs or foods or if you've got a vitamin or mineral deficiency, you are hindering the healing process.

What you can do to help it along is take better care of yourself. Get involved in your own care. Listen to your doctor, and to your body, but don't just listen to anyone, indiscriminately. What many of the best self-care and self-healing books, workshops and courses springing up all over the country do is help make you aware of what's happening to your own body. This doesn't mean, of course, that a broken leg, which normally takes six weeks to heal, can be willed into taking only three weeks. No. Most of the information on the art—and science—of self-care and self-healing concerns stress-related diseases such as headache, backache, high blood pressure, insomnia, colitis, asthma, alcoholism and cancer. These books and courses were never intended to replace doctors, but the best of them can help you experience the remarkable power and control you may have over internal body states by introducing you to techniques of biofeedback, relaxation, stress reduction and so on.

This new, nondrug frontier in Western medicine that is just opening up ranges all the way from Jacobson's Progressive Relaxation exercises to ancient herbal remedies that you can whip up in your own blender, and includes hypnosis, visualization, dream therapy, biogenics, Dioenergetics, journal-keeping, energy awareness, Transcendental Meditation, acupressure, acupinch, acupuncture, rolfing, and much else.*

We should caution you. There are con artists in every profession, and some of what is available on the subject of self-care and self-healing may be worthless, fraudulent and downright harmful. Some of it, on the other hand, could help save your life. What is important is to choose your teachers carefully, and not let yourself get suckered into anything just because it's trendy or expensive or promises instant results. Learning to understand and care for your body takes time and study. Quick cures are suspect—though doctors are more and more in awe of what miracles the human mind can accomplish once it sets to work on its kindred spirit, the body. You'll find more information on this in Chapter 5.

"HOW LONG WILL IT TAKE TO HEAL, DOC?"

Patients are always asking their doctors this after they've come in with a pulled tendon, or a torn muscle, or a bad break. The usual answer depends on several things. First is the severity of the injury. A minor sprain may take a few days; a major one, a few months. A torn cartilage means surgery no matter who you are, and you'll be out of action for six or eight weeks at least; a fractured tibia may take six months to heal.

Healing can actually be slowed down if you are not careful, or do dumb things. Using heat on an injury right away is dumb. So is taking off a cast early because you're curious about what your scar looks like and you feel like scratching. And it is especially unbright to give in to the injury so completely you do nothing but sit around and mope all day, afraid to move the injured part or too lazy to try. You *can* help yourself get back to full function faster by learning to do proper rehabilitation exercises. Depending on the injury, that could mean squeezing a rubber ball, or exercising on a Cybex machine at a gym, or

---

*There's an intelligent and informative magazine, *Medical Self-Care,* originated by a Yale Medical School graduate, Tom Ferguson, for the purpose of demystifying medicine and keeping people well and well-informed. Last time we checked, yearly subscriptions were available by writing him at P.O. Box 718, Inverness, California 94937.

practicing simple isometrics. The important thing is to be working toward rebuilding your muscle and restoring your arm or leg or shoulder to a full range of pain-free motion. If you're *not* working toward that, you're actually slowing down recovery time.

Another factor involved in healing is your mental attitude. If you tend to be a bitter, depressed, unpleasant person, chances are you will take much longer in getting back to tennis after a torn Achilles tendon than another player who takes his injury in stride, and pushes to keep going. The patients who seem to recover the fastest from sports injuries are strong-minded, positive-thinking men and women who want very much to get back to their sport. They are motivated.

After Wilt Chamberlain tore his quadriceps tendon a few years ago, early in the season, medical experts were astounded when he was back on the court in time for the playoffs. With that kind of injury, you'd expect him to be out for the year. Wilt was motivated. If Wanda the working wife, or Joe the assembly line worker suffered the same injury, it could be months before either would feel up to work again. The mind plays a tremendous role in healing, and if yours isn't working positively for you, it is working against you.

Finally, if you want to keep healing time to a minimum and playing time to a maximum, stay in condition and eat right. A fit body will feel ready to return to action faster than a tired, flabby, out-of-shape body. A body that is fueled on too much junk and deprived of proper nutrients will not heal as rapidly as one that is fed properly.

GETTING BACK TO PLAY: REHABILITATION

Too many recreational injuries are reinjuries. The acute pain goes away and you decide to try again even though you're not fully healed. Whether you go to a doctor or not, it is your responsibility to see to it that you are fully rehabilitated following any injury, no matter what it is, before you play again.

How do you know when you can play again? It is simple: when you can perform every motion and function that the sport requires normally and without pain. At least that's the ideal. This may vary somewhat from patient to patient. Highly motivated athletes may want to return to their sport though some pain is still with them, and in many instances that may be a perfectly reasonable thing to do. It depends on the injury, and the doctor, and how anxious the patient is to keep going. With every injury you get some temporary loss of function, however, and a returning athlete needs to be aware of what has happened to his body as a result of injuring it. Disuse usually leads to some atrophy or shrinking of the muscles, along with weakness, loss of motion and loss of flexibility. And as long as there is swelling you won't be able to regain free motion in the joint.

Ice and range-of-motion exercises help to reduce the swelling and increase the motion, and that's the first thing you need to do on your road to recovery. Next, you should work to regain the flexibility of the muscles that control the joint. A player with a chronically weak knee needs to strengthen the quadriceps and the hamstrings—the two major muscle groups that help keep his knee stable. If you've pulled a hamstring, you don't have to wait until it stops hurting to start getting the muscle back in shape. Work on it, but don't run on it until you've regained full strength and flexibility.

When you've got normal flexibility (see Chapter 7), work on strength (Chapter 8). Weak muscles are liable to be hurt again. Finally, when you've done everything there is to be done to get back flexibility and strength, work on functional activities: run, stop, change directions, jump—do all the things you have to do when you play. But when you go back to playing, do it gradually. If you've been off for ten weeks with a knee operation, don't expect to play the way you did the day you slammed into the backwall and tore the cartilage. Come back slowly and sensibly.

PILLS, SHOTS AND DRUGS

Drugs and sports will always be a subject of concern so long as there are people out there who want to run faster, jump higher, throw farther, heal faster—and other people willing to sell them a quick and easy solution. We can clear this issue up in no time—achievement does not come in a bottle. Pills will not make you jump higher, run faster or whatever—even though you may in fact do just that after taking them. Their effect is psychological—which isn't to say it isn't real, but that in reality *you* are bringing on the effect, not the medication.

Drugs can control pain and reduce inflammation, but the big problem comes in deciding which medications are safe—and effective—and which ones aren't. This is a vast and complicated issue, but overall the best bet is to avoid *all* medicines if you can. Try other things first. Sometimes you can't avoid them, and shouldn't. But be aware of all your options first. Ask questions. Do some reading on your own.

When your doctor prescribes something, ask him what it is, why he thinks it will be helpful and what its side effects might be. Again, there's a fine line between wanting to know and being offensive; be civil, but hold onto your confidence. You're paying the bills; you may be entitled to more satisfaction than you're getting now. But don't confuse satisfaction with cure. Your doctor can't do the work that only you can do for yourself. He cannot make your wounds heal any faster. There are enzyme drugs on the market that claim to make your bruises heal faster (Chymoral and Ananase are two brand names), but they aren't worth the money. Let your bruises heal at their own rate. The body that is allowed to heal itself is the cheapest and best cure there is.

DRUGS FOR TENDINITIS

The question of drugs for treatment most often comes up with tendinitis, since it is such a common sports malady. As we've pointed out, it comes on slowly and heals even more slowly. The body may take a couple of years to heal, and that can be terribly frustrating. The healthiest attitude for you to take is simply to accept the fact you have the problem, commit yourself to making sure it doesn't happen again and wait it out. That would be nature's way . . . but unfortunately, that isn't human nature. When you're hurt, angry and frustrated, you don't want a lecture on the Zen of sports medicine, you want help. You probably won't be satisfied if your doctor doesn't do *something*. One of David's medical partners, Dr. Bates Noble, is convinced that half the prescriptions that are written aren't filled. The patient feels better, though, just to have been given something.

What *something* can you be given for tendinitis, then? One of the best drugs doesn't require a prescription. It's aspirin, and it does several things. It's a good pain reliever; more than that, it is a good anti-inflammatory agent. All of the drugs available for tendinitis are anti-inflammatory agents, designed to combat the inflammation that naturally occurs when your body responds to all those microscopic tears that probably caused the tendinitis in the first place. The inflammation is actually the first stage of the healing process . . . a medical truism that may help you look more kindly on inflammation next time you have it. Unfortunately, with inflammation comes swelling, and it's the swelling that hurts. Anti-inflammatory agents reduce this reaction and therefore the symptoms. The acetylsalicylic acid component that constitutes aspirin (as well as Bufferin, Excedrin, Anacin and so on) is the active ingredient that works against inflammation. Since this ingredient is missing from the popular pain-killing Tylenol, it won't do much against inflammation.

Other drugs your doctor might prescribe include Butazolidin, Indocin, Motrin, Tolectin or Naprosyn. They are more potent than the lowly aspirin.

WHAT ABOUT CORTISONE?

Cortisone is an artificial hormone that was discovered some thirty years ago. It is probably the most potent of all the available anti-inflammatory agents. But like all the others, it can have serious side effects: it can upset your stomach, cause rashes, affect your blood count, make you retain fluid or harm your liver, among other problems. Cortisone once looked promising for patients crippled by bursitis and arthritis, but it is now known to cause more side effects than any other anti-inflammatory drug. You can take aspirin for a longer period of time than any other drug; but it too can cause problems. Some people, and David is one of them, develop allergic reactions to it.

So, caught between a rock and a hard place, what's a patient to do? Most of the drugs your doctor might prescribe, even cortisone, can usually be used safely for short periods of time. If you don't get significantly good results in about five days, you might as well flush the pills away and try something, or someone, else. Taking more drugs, longer, won't make your problem any better . . . and it could make you feel a lot worse. If you are going to stay on the anti-inflammatory drugs for more than five days, be sure to get directions from your doctor about things to watch for. He should be watching your blood count, and you should be watching for any unusual signs or symptoms of something wrong. If your body throws up a red alert, or even a mildly pink one, stop taking the medicine.

As for the cortisone shots, though they certainly are popular among ailing athletes, more and more their safety is being questioned. A serious player with a terrible tendinitis or red-hot shoulder bursitis can get amazingly quick and efficient pain relief from an injection with hydrocortisone, a derivative of cortisone, and the drug has a place in treatment, *if* the patient is informed and can find relief from nothing else, or *if* the pain is severe to the point of being disabling. But now that the use of cortisone-like steroids has developed into a $225-million business, doctors have to be careful not to abuse the drug, or the patient, by cavalierly prescribing this treatment. Indeed, it should not be used in a particular tendon more than two, or at most three, times a year. Be extremely cautious about allowing shots in major tendons such as the patellar or Achilles tendon. There is no question that the drug will cause some temporary change in the structure of the tendon. Although it may reduce your symptoms, ease your pain, and after a few days' rest allow you to get back on the playing field, it also knocks out one of the body's important warning signs. And continued heavy use of the tendon—more running, jumping and so on—may actually cause the altered tendon to rupture. If you can avoid cortisone altogether you're much better off.

CAN'T RELAX? YOU'RE BETTER OFF MEDITATING THAN MEDICATING

Muscle relaxants are another kind of drug frequently prescribed for sports-related injuries. When you're hurt, you may feel nervous, tense, anxious. You need to relax, and rest, but you can't settle down. Muscle relaxants work like tranquilizers; they artificially induce you to do what you can easily learn to do for yourself: quiet the mind and body by means of biofeedback training, deep relaxation exercises or other awareness routines. But again, too often patients are looking for instant relief from anxiety, and too often doctors are willing to give in to their demands for an easy way out. Pill abuse is a serious, debilitating epidemic in this country. One hundred million prescriptions a year are written for tranquilizers, allowing Americans to down at least 4 billion Valium and Librium pills annually. Such drug abuse is crippling and costly in terms of lives lost and money wasted.

You can enrich your own life and save yourself a lot of aggravation by avoiding the mind-numbing tranquilizers altogether. If you want to alter your consciousness, you're much better off running slowly for an hour or swimming laps for a mile. Fitness really can help your psyche if you stick with it: it can calm you down, perk you up and make you much better able to cope with life. Tranquilizers promise that, but they don't deliver in the long run. You're a million times better off getting hooked on running than running through life hooked on uppers and downers, with Valiums in between. But you know that already, don't you? What you may not know is that regular exercise may help you get unhooked. The natural high you can get from slow, long-distance workouts can negate your need to pop, inject, snort, smoke, drink or otherwise artifically sedate or stimulate yourself. Self-care doesn't mean abstinence from the pleasures of life, but it can help you rediscover the pleasure *in* life—in health, in feeling your fittest.

WHAT ABOUT X-RAYS?

Many people are becoming concerned about X-rays and their bad effects. We don't blame them. No one can tolerate too many X-rays—but how many is too many? It's easy to look at the nation-at-large and say that we are over-X-rayed and overmedicated, but when it boils down to an individual injured party—to you and your painful arm in the emergency room of the nearest hospital, fresh from a collision between your bike and a high curb—it's unrealistic to talk about treatment before getting a complete set of X-rays. It's almost impossible to tell the difference between a sprain and a fracture without one. If you are certain that your sports accident involves only a pulled muscle, then an X-ray isn't necessary. But if you are a runner complaining of foot pain or shin splints, you will need an X-ray so that your doctor can at least eliminate the possibility of a congenital problem or a stress fracture. In any ailment where diagnosis is difficult—back pain, for example—you can expect a lot of X-rays. With back pain, it's necessary to make sure that your problem doesn't stem from a worn disc or a congenital abnormality or some kind of wear change that could affect your treatment or recovery time.

Most doctors will also take an X-ray when you come in complaining of tendinitis. Even though the condition is probably as we've described it, and even though it will get better if just left alone, it's probably wise to find out whether there are any calcium deposits or whether you've pulled off any flecks of bone from the tendon attachment.

X-rays are valuable tools and a necessary evil of modern medicine. If you don't want to have any taken, don't get hurt.

COPING WITH PAIN

Very often, self-care for injuries boils down to two things: developing patience and dealing with pain. We've talked about the patience part as a positive mental attitude, the confidence that this too shall pass. Dealing with the pain of a sports injury can be a very trying and frustrating experience, especially when you understand that pain pills or shots are not really the answer. To be your own best answer, you will need to learn about some of the newer, nondrug ways of coping with pain. There is a Pain Rehabilitation Clinic in LaCrosse, Wisconsin, for instance, run by Dr. Norman Shealy, whose patients learn to control pain by relaxing their bodies and focusing their minds through autogenic training and biofeedback. Dr. Shealy describes his program of stress control, which he calls Biogenics, in a book, *90 Days to Self Health.*

One thing that helps in coping with pain is the security of knowing where the pain is coming from and when it might be leaving.

I-C-E and aspirin can help you cope; so can stretching and relaxation. Panic, on the other hand, makes pain worse. A good way to calm down and avoid panicking at the first twinge of pain is a few good deep breaths. Don't give in to the pain or let it get the best of you. Make up your mind that you will control the pain, that it will not control you. Deep breathing, relaxation, visualization can all help get your body-mind in harmony, and help you get the upper hand. (There is more about this in Chapter 5.) Runners who used to be stymied by the pain of a stitch or muscle cramp, for instance, now find they can work through the pain by practicing the sort of deep-breathing exercises that have been taught in Lamaze natural childbirth classes for years. You can take those same principles—of relaxation, selective concentration, blowing out air through pursed lips and so on—and apply them to any sport or to any pain. Your reward for working out ways to cope with pain is that you're able to keep going. And that's one of the most important factors in achieving fitness—just to keep going. You do have to be careful, though. You mustn't forget that pain *can* be an important warning signal. How do you tell the difference between pain-you-run-through and pain-you-pay-attention-to? You don't; your body does. The more in tune with it you are, the better care you can give it.

WOMEN AND SELF-CARE

For too long, women were discouraged from participating in sports. They're having to play catch-up ball now, but they are making tremendous strides forward, and the prospect of women's full and welcome participation in sports looks bright. But nagging bits of medical misinformation still linger on, scaring women away, making them think that they are risking their lives, their limbs, their femininity if they pursue fitness too vigorously. All nonsense. Of course there are risks involved when you run, or play tennis, or shoot baskets. But these exist for *all* athletes. Women need to be as cautious as any sensible male athlete, but there's no reason to think that they are significantly more prone to injury.

What about special equipment? Should women take special care to protect their breasts in collision sports such as basketball or rugby? *All* players need adequate protection for their sport—e.g., eyeguards for racquetball, shin pads for volleyball and so on. Women don't require any extra swaddling clothes. In fact, it's men, not women, who need to be concerned about protecting the genital area with plastic cup devices. Title IX funds will never have to be spent on anything like a Jill Strap. Nor do women need to take extra precautions to protect their breasts. No one likes a blow to the chest—and if it's serious enough, it may in fact raise a bump or cause a bruise. But the old wives' tale that women who get hit in the breasts stand a greater chance of getting cancer is pure superstition. The only time breasts are a problem is in sports like running, when all the flopping and bouncing can lead to pain and torn tissue. In the last year, several name-brand manufacturers have come out with sport bras designed to be supportive, but not binding or uncomfortable. Women athletes ought to be able to find a style that suits them, or they can resort to the old-fashioned, low-cost alternative of simply wrapping a 6-inch elastic bandage around their chest a few times. It's not the most attractive solution but it does serve the purpose.

HEAT, COLD AND ALTITUDE

If you're going to be exercising in a climate that is very hot, very cold or very high, there are some special precautions you should take. The problem in working out when it's very warm is that you increase the risk of heat injuries. If your body can't keep cool and your core temperature rises, you can collapse and die. In Chapter 6, on nutrition, we'll talk about this serious overheating problem in detail. For now, you should understand your responsibility for taking care of your own needs when you're exercising where it's hot. Drink plenty of fluids before, during and after activity. If you are playing and feel woozy or nauseous or out of sorts, don't push on. Listen to your body and respect it. The better condition you're in, the better able to tolerate the heat you'll be. If you are looking toward a summer golf or tennis tournament, or a long midday run, you should acclimate yourself to the heat little by little. Wear sport clothes that absorb moisture and let your skin breathe. (Cotton is usually better in this regard than polyester blends.) Don't tough it out and refuse to drink fluids while you're exercising. That macho philosophy can kill you.

Hypothermia—getting too cold—is a killer too, and you'd be surprised how easy it is to have your body temperature drop down to fatal or near-fatal temperatures. Winter runners, skiers, outdoor swimmers and any others whose sport exposes them to the elements need to be aware what a dangerous game they are playing when they play outdoors in the cold. The first line of defense is to dress wisely and warmly. Several thin layers will trap your body heat and keep you more comfortable than one thick layer. The more wool involved the better, though we've seen steam-breathing runners out on below-freezing days, running in little more than a cotton sweat suit. Vigorous exercise will warm you up. What you should wear depends on your tolerance for cold, and on the vigorousness of your sport. If you're going out to ice-fish at 10° above you might as well dredge up every warm item you have. If you're planning a 10-mile cross-country ski trip, the chances are that you can strip down to jeans and a flannel shirt and still feel toasty warm. It's important to keep your hands and your feet protected (extremities are prime candidates for frostbite) and it's especially smart to wear a hat, since anywhere from 50 to 70 percent of your body heat can escape out the top of an uncovered head.

Winter sports enthusiasts are always wondering if it's bad for them to expose themselves to the cold weather. It might be uncomfortable at first, if you haven't gradually gotten used to the change in climate, but if you're reasonably cautious, the cold weather won't hurt you. It certainly can't freeze your lungs—as some runners fear. Dress warm, use a face mask if the cold is too biting and protect your face and lips from raw winds with cream or vaseline. Be sure to warm up your muscles before you start any hard pounding, and when you're through running, get your sweaty body indoors as soon as possible. Avoid chills. Avoid ice, too, since the greatest danger of winter running probably comes from misstepping on ice, or sidestepping a patch of snow. If it's too cold for you to be comfortable running, you're better off working up a sweat some other way, since a body that is tense and shivering is prone to injury.

Altitude sickness isn't exactly a sports injury, but it does affect great numbers of skiers, backpackers, climbers and other athletes who pursue their sport in the high reaches of the atmosphere. The higher you go, the thinner the air, the less oxygen there is and the harder your heart has to work to keep you in proper working condition. Fortunately, our bodies adapt to changes in altitude pretty fast . . . though not as rapidly as we'd like sometimes. In the meantime, altitude sickness can leave us feeling tired, nauseous and out of breath, with a pounding headache. The best way to avoid any problems is to give your body a couple of days to adjust itself to the higher altitude before you ask it to perform. If you're skiing Telluride this year, don't take a plane out in the morning and expect to conquer The Plunge in the afternoon. Also, be sure and drink plenty of fluids since any degree of dehydration will make the symptoms even worse.

II. Keep Going

5. Mental

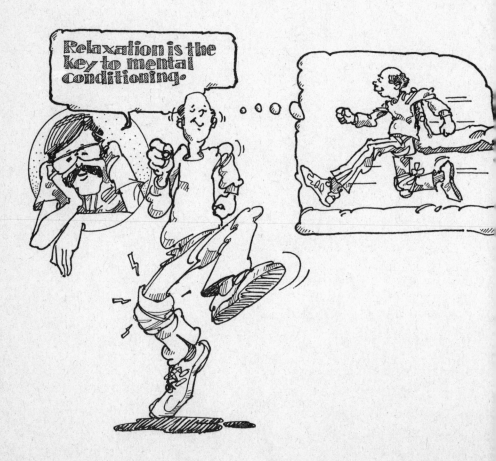

Conditioning

Dear Dr. Jock:

I read in People magazine that the movie actress Cicely Tyson meditates before she runs and that just because she does that, she's able to run 10 miles or more. I don't see what one has to do with the other, do you? I guess I'm asking because I've tried twice to get a running program started and each time I got so bored with it I just had to quit. Maybe I should meditate, too. What does meditation have to do with it anyhow? And how does something you do in your head work so good on your feet?

T.F., Greenville, South Carolina

Dear Dr. Jock:

I'm not a runner but a lot of my friends are. In the warm weather I play basketball and tennis and in the winter go cross-country skiing a lot. Here's what I'm wondering: I hear my friends all the time talking about getting high when they run. You know what I mean. They'll be running and after maybe an hour, sometimes they'll feel like they're just floating along the road. I feel that same way sometimes when I go skiing. Not all the time, but when I do, it's real neat. What is that feeling? Why do we get it? Is there such a thing as getting it too much? Is it ever dangerous?

L.F., Buffalo, New York

Dear Dr. Jock:

I play golf with a guy I've known for fifteen years. We were buddies in the Army together and we both work at the same company now. He's a good friend of mine and I trust him. But he read in a book, or a magazine, something about visualization and tried to explain to me how it's helped his game a whole lot because now, before he hits the ball, he first thinks about what it looks like but then when he gets up to actually hit the ball, he doesn't think at all. I don't understand what he's talking about but meanwhile his game is getting better and I'm in a real slump.

*What is this visualization stuff about and how does it work? (Please
don't use my name in the paper.)*

A.J., Elyria, Ohio

Jim is a copy editor for a national magazine. He's in his thirties,
handsome, something of a ladykiller, and before he started running he
was close to 20 pounds overweight. The first time he ran he was so out
of shape he thought he'd die, but after two tough weeks he conquered
his first mile and hasn't stopped since. He loves running, loves the way
it makes him feel, loves the afterglow. His only problem is occasional
knee pain. He'd wrenched his knee playing football in college and even
though he did his stretching routine regularly, he'd sometimes feel his
knee tighten up and begin to hurt just ten minutes into his run. He
tried different shoes, a $150 orthotic and softer turf, but nothing
seemed to help. Jim checked with his doctor to be sure he wasn't
making his knee any worse by running, and was left to deal with the
discomfort or quit running—a thought that actually made him wake
up nights in a cold sweat.

One day his friend Roberta told him about a trick she'd learned from
a remarkable lady who travels around the country, talking about the
yin and yang of body awareness, about using sport to transcend
physical limitations, about everyday athletes reaching toward magical
spaces of ecstasy and oneness with the Universe. Her name is Dyveke
Spino, and her New Age approach to coaching isn't new really. Nor is it
limited to running.

What Roberta picked up from Dyveke and passed on to Jim really
isn't a trick at all. To begin the process, Roberta suggested that the
next time Jim was out running and felt that tired, testy cramp in his
knee beginning to come on, instead of slowing down or tightening up,
he should simply relax. It sounds simple, but the truth is that really
getting the body to relax is the hardest part of the exercise; usually,
the more we tell ourselves to relax, the tenser we get. Roberta knew all
about this; she'd had a habit she couldn't break of running with her
shoulders hunched, so that on a long run the tension in her neck really
took its toll. But then she signed up for some sessions in biofeedback
and in an hour or two on her doctors' sensitive machines she learned
how to focus awareness on those tight neck muscles and unlock the
tension. Now, every day, she does 15 minutes of deep relaxation (a
form of meditation) and 15 minutes of yoga stretches. She's never felt
better. With the neck pain gone, Roberta is free to enjoy her running as
never before. In no time at all, she doubled her distance from 4 to 8
miles and shaved a full 5 minutes off her best time.

Jim thought the whole relaxation-visualization thing sounded
far-out, but since nothing else seemed to work, he agreed to go along

with Roberta's suggestions about how to relax. When you feel the pain, she said, instead of telling yourself how much it hurts and what a relief it would be to stop running, try and sink yourself, your thoughts, your awareness down to your knee and feel around it until you can visualize the pain. Is it hot or cold? Red or yellow? Tingly or dull? Above the kneecap or inside it? Once you've got your mind focused on your knee, once you've taken inventory of what a sore knee looks like, of precisely how it feels, the next thing to do is to think of something that would make it feel better, and then apply it mentally. What about hundreds of tiny hands gently massaging away the pain? Or perhaps a cool waterfall that starts at the top of your head and flows effortlessly down through your entire body, washing all the tension out of your arms and legs and making your knee feel especially nice? It doesn't matter what the fantasy is, Roberta said, or the sport, for that matter, so long as it works for you. As Jim listened, it sounded weird—too weird for anyone who scrupulously avoided even knowing his astrological sign. But Jim was desperate.

So one time he tried a little fantasy. It was a very little one, and he didn't tell a soul about it for months; but whenever he'd be out running and he'd feel his knee begin to tighten, the first thing he'd do was shake loose. It was his way—until he learned a better one—of relaxing. He'd just run along and let his arms dangle, and his head and shoulders flop. Sometimes, if he felt like it, he'd make burgle-gurgle noises with his mouth. ("Sounds are good," Roberta had told him— "good for the breathing and good for the soul.") Whatever he did, Jim could feel it loosening him up. But still he had an agonizing knee pain to cope with. Then he'd get a mental picture of his knee, of how red and bloated it looked, how hot and throbbing it felt; and then he thought about running—not on his knee, but on two big, soft pillows, or two balloons—and now every time Jim stepped down, he could visualize himself lightly bouncing back up. When he did that, his stride eased and he began to float down the running path—pain-free. That sensation of floating helped him forget all about his knee. Besides which, it was a real high for Jim. Sometimes he'd conjure up that same flotation fantasy whether or not his knee was hurting, purely for the pleasure of it.

THE BODY AND THE MIND ARE ONE

We're not saying that visualization is the panacea for all your sports aches and pains. But the story of Jim and Roberta is typical of what's happening in this country, as more and more smart athletes come to grips with the fact that physical aches and pains can be helped or heightened by what's going on in your mind. They are discovering—in books, in workshops, through body-mind disciplines like yoga, or the

Alexander technique, or bioenergetics, or rolfing or (not often enough) through their own doctors—that the mind and the body are inscrutably, inextricably linked, and that what you do with your mind while running, or skiing, or playing tennis, very much affects the way your body performs.

The reverse is also true, of course: the body affects the mind. People who fight the good fight to get physically fit report experiencing a real surge in emotional fitness. Call it a rush, a high, a flow, a glow—regular, vigorous exercise can bring on these waves of well-being. It can enhance your creativity, help you think more clearly. Robert Merrill, the singer, actually meditates when he runs: "I just listen to my legs and feet, turn everything off, and my mind becomes very clear."

All this talk about relaxation, visualization, meditation and the body-mind connection may have sounded like hokum ten years ago, when barefoot prophets wearing gauze shirts and Phi Beta Kappa keys first started talking about body awareness. All that talk—about listening to your body's inner voices, about the harmonious rhythms of the fine-tuned body-mind—was the sort of cosmic thinkspeak that California is known for, and that people who pride themselves on being logical try to ignore. But biofeedback made the body-mind impossible to ignore in the early 70s, and the word got out—in the last few years of the fitness boom, especially—that being in touch with your body meant something after all. It wasn't just jargon, it was a way of being. It meant a release of tension, a sense of calm, more energy and less flab.

Some people still have a hard time accepting it. One biofeedback pioneer, Dr. Barbara Brown, explains the problem this way:

> The concept about biofeedback that we Americans find so difficult to believe is that some totally unconscious yet complex sophisticated mental process might be "supermind," that we may actually possess mental capabilities that can absorb information about internal states and use that information to bring internal functioning up to an optimum level. We find such a concept difficult to believe because our philosophy and our psychology say that to achieve anything, to conquer anything, takes effort, consciously directed hard work. We believe that we can't be productive unless we keep concentrating on our goals, attending, consciously directing our actions. Yet apparently the trick in biofeedback is to get the consciousness out of the picture, let the information pour in and let whatever mental giant resides in the great unconsciousness use that information to put our body's activities aright without conscious interference. It's part of the process Dr. Elmer Green (and Schultz before him) calls passive volition, or the process the free spirits use when they say, "Let it happen," and put their conscious awareness and direction and interference aside to let the good things happen.

More and more, people are learning to let the good things happen. All across the country, runners, walkers, skiers, tennis players, hikers, martial artists, racquetball players, swimmers and many millions of other recreational athletes have begun to rediscover their bodies. Working out, regular exercise, endurance sports have become ways to transform your self, your body, your entire personality.

Relaxation, meditation, deep breathing, visualization are only a few of the new techniques that can help you make that transformation for yourself. Indeed, they are only a small part of an exciting body-mind revolution that is changing the thinking—and the training—of some doctors and of many active, athletic people like you.

A BALANCED BODY-MIND IS CRUCIAL IN SPORTS

The deeper we delve into the miracles of the body, the more likely we are to emerge talking about the mysteries of the mind. No getting around that, because it's all connected. Mind really matters when it comes to sports and exercise, and mind-over-matter can mean the difference between finishing the marathon and quitting at the Wall, six miles short. It can mean powerhousing your normally mild-mannered forehand past the Incredible Hulk across the net, or making it down the most mogul-monstrous run of the day, tired but still standing.

The more understanding you have of the connections between your body and your mind, the better you'll be as an athlete. The more aware you are of your body's own natural ability to heal itself, the more alert you are to signs your body is wearing down, the more you tune in to your body's deep inner voice and learn to influence what it says, the better you'll be able to perform.

Too often, when you hear about sports performance and injury prevention, you hear only about the physical. You hear about strength, flexibility, oxygen uptake and pulse, and you may forget that for every hard, measurable physical parameter of fitness there is a softer, subtler aspect waiting to be dealt with—the mental one. The body influences the mind and vice versa.

A healthy person, then—according to holistic theory—is one whose total body-mind system is in balance. The 17th-century French philosopher René Descartes thought otherwise, and Western doctors who picked up on his theories view the mind as separate and distinct from the body. Traditional Western medicine does not regard the individual as a psychobiological unit. Unlike the more ancient traditions of the East, it does not view the patient as a complex being whose thoughts, perceptions, anxieties, fears and memories are intimately linked to chemistry, biology and physiology. It merely treats disease. It deals in cures, not prevention. While modern-day psychiatrists and psychologists treat the mind, a host of other medical specialists divvy up the body, and the twain rarely meet.

However, times are changing. Old beliefs are giving way to irrefutable new evidence and new ways of healing. Nowadays, even the most conservative Western doctors will admit that between 50 and 80 percent of all the so-called body ailments and diseases they see have been influenced, and sometimes clearly caused, by the patient's emotional state. Less conservative physicians say 100 percent. They believe everything that affects a patient affects a patient's health—that all diseases are psychosomatic. That doesn't mean the pain isn't "real"—or that the patient is "pretending." No, psychosomatic illness hurts just the same as the real thing. Only the cause of the pain isn't in the body as much as it is in the mind. Pain control, then, is very often mind control—which helps explain why patients often feel so much relief after learning to release tension, or taking a placebo, or visiting an alternative healer.

Faith and hope and a positive mental attitude have a powerful effect on the body's own natural healing processes. We see this all the time in sports medicine. Two individuals who suffer similar sports injuries may experience very different healing histories, depending in large part on their mental attitudes and on how much responsibility they're willing to assume for their own health and well-being.

For too long, Western medicine has denied patients the responsibility. Doctors have treated them mechanically, like a body to be healed instead of a body-mind capable of healing itself. When we help patients understand how much power they have to help themselves, we can, hopefully, help them choose wellness over sickness. The important thing is that they recognize they have a choice.

VIGOROUS EXERCISE CAN WORK WONDERS ON YOUR MIND

Although a balanced, healthy mind won't guarantee you a healthy, injury-free body, it can certainly play a significant role. We already know that regular, vigorous exercise frequently has a positive effect on the mind. Dr. Thaddeus Kostrubala, author of *The Joy of Running*, has become famous for treating his psychiatric patients on the run. There's a marathon-running shrink in Chicago named Dr. Shelly Greenberg, who is just as high on his version of LSD—Long, Slow Distance running—to help hard-core cases break out of their self-destructive habits.

The running craze has left us inspirational stories the way Johnny Appleseed left us apple trees—testimonials from born-again runners about how running can boost self-esteem, alleviate depression, bring on dreams, spark creativity and boost sexual prowess (or at least desire). Women athletes, especially late-blooming runners, have been very vocal about the strength and confidence they feel from sports, once they've gotten past their fear of trying. Why all this happens hasn't really been nailed down. There are several theories.

Some researchers think a vigorous exercise like running is a natural turn-on to the production of norepinephrine, a natural chemical in the brain that helps make important links between the neurons. Depression can be a problem with people who are deficient in norepinephrine, so regular exercise may give them a way to boost their production of it *without* the nasty side effects and the national scandal of all those antidepressant drugs and pills.

Another explanation for the mind benefits of fitness comes from researchers concerned with chronic migraine and cluster headaches, who find that the excruciating pain and pressure can sometimes be curbed in as little as five minutes of running. Doctors theorize that the vigorous workout and endurance training may prompt the body to produce a particular enzyme to prevent blood vessels in the brain from expanding and causing grief when they press against the nerves.

Some psychiatrists believe that too much salt in the body can lead to depression. Another of the biological benefits of vigorous exercise, then, is that it causes you to sweat away some of that excess salt. This may be why some women who suffer miserably from "menstrual bloat blues" have found relief in regular exercise. The less salt, the less water retention, and the better they feel.

Another interesting theory is suggested by Dr. Phillip Nuernberger at the Center for Stress Management and Research of the Himalayan Institute in Honesdale, Pennsylvania, where a lot of research is being done on breath control. He suggests that runners who inhale and exhale out of the nose (the best breathing method for average speeds) may experience winds of up to 200 mph rushing in through the nostrils. This is very stimulating to the nose's highly sensitive receptors, and may well account for the mysterious "runners' high."

Of course, vigorous exercise also makes us feel good for the very obvious reason that it pumps more adrenaline into the system, circulates more glucose and helps deliver bigger and better wallops of oxygen and blood to the brain. In some instances, all this increased activity may even help the right brain—the more intuitive, creative side—assert itself over the more rational, logical left brain. The result may be those creative flashes and mesmerizing highs athletes have lately been tantalizing us with.

CALL IT WHAT YOU WILL, BUT LEARN TO GO WITH THE FLOW

If you can find a way to make the workout rewarding in and of itself, you've found the secret of how to keep going. That's always the goal for a recreational athlete, but sometimes it's hard to pin down how so much pleasure can be derived from something that can also bring so much pain. A researcher at the University of Chicago, Mihaly Csikszentmihalyi, has come up with a concept he calls Flow. By Flow he means that feeling of buoyancy and strength you get when you're bicycling down a country road at a steady 20 mph, when the sun is out and the road is clear. It's the feeling that runners can't stop talking about even when they know how overzealous they sound, the feeling of freedom from pressure, freedom to experience the rhythm of one's own life. It's the satisfaction you feel when you're doing anything that makes you feel utterly in tune with yourself and at peace with the world.

Flow is one of the New Age words for what the old-time athletes wouldn't talk about out loud. Men who were brought up conditioned to think of sports competition as another version of the "Mine Is Bigger than Yours" game sometimes have a hard time enjoying their sport, finding their flow. They tend to be too competitive, too wrapped up in the idea that for sports to be good, someone's gotta get hurt.

Women may experience a block of the opposite kind when they first start working out, running, lifting weights, shooting baskets or perfecting that kill shot from eight feet back of the line. They have to get over their fears of appearing too butch, too athletic, too muscular. Once they do that, they get into the flow and discover the indescribable pleasure of exercise, quite apart from the extrinsic rewards of firming up mottled flesh and beefing up a flaccid heart.

A lot of people in this country are fitness dropouts. They may resolve to keep exercising after the 10 pounds are off and the summer bikini is packed away, but only a small percentage really do. There's hope that the percentage will grow as more and more people experience the relation between regular exercise and the quality of their lives, emotionally as well as physically.

THE SPIRITUAL UNDERGROUND IN SPORTS IS NOW WELL DOCUMENTED

Top athletes are now beginning to speak out about the moments of ecstasy and transcendence they sometimes feel when they're sprinting at top speed in the 100-yard dash, or slam-dunking perfect baskets, or hurtling around corners at speeds up to 200 mph. Consciousness is altered, perception is distorted. Time stands still. Past lives may emerge, future events become predictable. The marathon swimmer Diana Nyad said before she attempted to swim from Cuba to Miami that her biggest fear was of losing touch with reality altogether. How close to the edge could she come in a 60-hour swim and still get safely back to shore?

Michael Murphy and Rhea White have collaborated on a fascinating book, *The Psychic Side of Sports*, which documents extraordinary psychic events in sports—including ESP, psychokinetic and out-of-body experiences, as well as many exceptional feats of strength and endurance. They write, "The many reports we have collected (some 4500) show us that sport has enormous power to sweep us beyond the ordinary sense of self, to evoke capacities that have generally been regarded as mystical, occult, or religious." They haven't come up with a precise formula for achieving such moments, nor do they pretend that all athletes are closet mystics. However, they have come up with one thing that can be extremely useful to recreational athletes: "Regardless of the sport, successful athletes say that when they are performing at their best they are immersed in the present moment, totally involved in what confronts them."

In the same book, former San Francisco Forty-Niner quarterback, John Brodie, is quoted as saying, "A player's effectiveness is directly related to his ability to be right there, doing that thing, in the moment. All the preparation he may have put into the game—all the game plans, analysis of movies, etc.—is no good if he can't put it into action when game time comes. He can't be worrying about the past or the future or the crowd or some other extraneous event. He must be totally able to respond in the here and now."

Tim Gallwey calls this playing "the inner game." You can do it once you learn to stop nagging yourself during a game ("Keep that left arm straight!" "Dummy!" "What if I lose?"). You'll also cut down the risk of injury because the less tense you are, the less vulnerable your body is to strains, sprains and those tiny rips from overuse that lead to tendinitis.

YOU CAN LEARN TO HANDLE STRESS

Everyone is under some stress, but few people really know how to cope with it. Stress is that proverbial double-edged sword: we need some of it to know we are alive, to feel stretched and strong and confident. But too much stress, inadequately dealt with, is one of the most destructive forces in day-to-day living. Stress makes us sick. It can kill if we let it defeat us. Stress is a factor in heart attacks, ulcers, strokes, headaches, backaches, arthritis, respiratory diseases such as bronchitis, and many others, including cancer. If you ask a doctor what percentage of the patients he sees have stress-related ailments, and he gives an honest answer, he'll say 70 percent or more. Have you asked yourself what you are doing to cope with the stress in your life? You can't avoid it and if you refuse to deal with it consciously, those unrelieved tensions may creep into your unconscious, worm into the functioning of your body and eventually wear it down. In the words of Hans Selye, the world-famous authority on stress and disease, "If you use too much of your energy in resisting the stresses and strains of life, it's like running your car through the streets and keeping your brakes on at the same time. You will wear it out much more rapidly."

Unrelieved stress takes its toll in sports performance too. The pros have to learn how to handle it, just as you do. One way, of course, is to ask a doctor for drugs to relax the muscles and ease tension—but we've already harped enough on how this way has been abused. There also are a variety of body-mind disciplines for relieving stress—including rolfing, Feldenkreis, bioenergetics and the Alexander technique, among others. They're all geared to freeing the body's flow of energy. Underlying them all is the theme that there is a constant flow of energy between body and mind—between physiology and psychology—and that when the flow is blocked or whacked out of balance, there is a problem. The problem could be physical—a headache, a backache or an ulcer—or it could be an emotional one, showing up as anxiety, fear or depression. The block could cause bad posture or a twisted knee. Most body therapists won't dwell on *why* your body isn't performing at its peak; they concentrate on helping you understand how you can overcome the problem and perform better. Whereas a hard-core Freudian analyst may not sleep at night until he is certain that your habit of running on your toes is the outcome of early toilet training, body-mind therapists don't dwell on the past. For them, a body problem is a body awareness problem.

Bioenergeticists, for instance, say that the first and biggest obstacle to the body's natural ability to heal itself is the patient's unawareness of the tensions in the body. Their aim is for people to learn what stress feels like, and then work to get rid of that stress. The Alexander technique helps people to overcome a variety of modern illnesses by retraining them to use their bodies gracefully, without tension. The less tension, the less stress, the less chance you have of disease or injury. Rolfing—a series of ten body-realignment sessions developed by Ida Rolf, Ph.D—attempts to reduce stress on the body by releasing contractions or constrictions in the connective tissue (fascia) so that the force of gravity works with the body instead of against it. Runners with a persistent foot and leg problem sometimes choose to go through the painful process of rolfing. Other athletes choose it, or any of the other body-mind disciplines, not because of a specific medical problem but simply in order to increase body awareness and learn more about the body's own natural ability to heal itself.

When you think about body-mind disciplines as a tool to educate people about their own bodies and get them tuned in to their own ability to prevent injury and disease and promote healing, the craziness from California begins to make sense. It also makes dollars-and-sense when you consider the runaway cost of medical care. Instead of National Health Insurance, what this country ought to have is a Health Assurance plan. If we had one, medical doctors would start assuring patients that the secret to good health is no secret at all, but a combination of eating the right foods, regular exercise, good genes and some means of dealing with the stress and tensions of everyday life. Self-help, self-care groups with this purpose are springing up, and if you're careful about choosing one and don't spend too much money in the process, joining one could be a good move for you.

A medical writer, Carol Kahn, once asked René Dubos, the famed bacteriologist who spent some fifty years at the Rockefeller Institute for Medical Research, about how the nation's health dollars could best be spent. He didn't mention hospitals, research and technology, or even increasing the number of medical schools. What he recommended was what the body-mind folks have been urging for years—education:

> I think a lot of money should be spent on convincing people that drugging yourself for everything that goes wrong is a silly way of taking care of your health. If a process of education could be found to convey to people that most of the things from which you suffer will be better by themselves and that most of the drugs you take don't help and many can harm, it would do much more good than a national health service.

CHOOSE YOUR SPORT CAREFULLY

Just because so many millions have taken up running doesn't mean it's the right sport for you. Your body may not be built to take the stresses involved. Your mind may more easily adjust to the rhythms of bicycling or swimming. Just walking can be good exercise too, if you step lively enough. The important thing is to find a way to enjoy whatever sport you choose, enough to experience that flow, that high, that shiver of good feeling. Once you've had that experience, the arrival of some mysterious ache or pain won't become a reason to stop working out. You'll look instead for ways to stop the hurting.

If you're the cause, you'll inquire into what emotional hurt you might be trying to work out. If it's a seemingly mechanical injury—a torn ligament, an Achilles tendinitis—you will be asking yourself what stress you've allowed to build up. You'll know that inflexible muscles cause 8 out of 10 sports injuries, and you'll come to grips with the necessity for spending more than 5 minutes, every other day, loosening up those tight muscles.

No one's looking to blame you for your pain or illness or injury. Your choice—if you chose at all—was most likely unconscious. All of us have a difficult time dealing with the stress in our life—you're not the only one. But once you begin to see yourself as a victim of your own unconscious choice, then you are halfway home to learning how to take better care of yourself.

"Prevention begins when we identify sources of stress, sensitize ourselves to crucial bodily signals, and take steps to reduce this stress," says Dr. Kenneth R. Pelletier, who wrote *Mind as Healer, Mind as Slayer* and is an expert on psychosomatic medicine. His point and our point too is that you can choose to deal with your stress in positive ways, in new ways, healthy ways. You don't have to keep it locked in, tied up with ribbons of guilt and trapped within tight, tense muscles. You can learn to reduce stress and get what it is you really want out of life without turning to sickness.

DON'T SET YOURSELF UP FOR FAILURE

Once you've settled on which sport is right for you, and you're committed to enjoying it to its fullest, be realistic about the level you begin playing it at.

"One prerequisite for flow is an even match between the difficulty of a challenge and a person's ability to meet it. If the demands are too slight, the person feels bored; if it is too great, he feels anxious," says Daniel Goleman, a Boulder, Colorado, therapist who has put out an instructional tape cassette called "Flow and Mindfulness." "Games lend themselves to flow because, unlike life itself, we can control their difficulty and adjust their challenge to fit our skills. The golfer changes his handicap, the tennis player chooses a partner of equal ability." Whatever you choose to play, don't be so tough on yourself you make it impossible to succeed. But don't underestimate your potential either. If you're a skier, choose a hill that will challenge you, but spend a little time visualizing your trip down, making sure that you have the skills and energy to run it safely.

If you're a mediocre racquetball player who is always getting beaten, and you feel blatantly inferior to your opponent, it is unlikely that you'll experience warm, flowing feelings about your sport.

RELAXATION IS THE KEY TO MENTAL CONDITIONING

To open up those feelings, you'll need to learn a technique for calming the chatter constantly going on in the mind. That doesn't mean you should try to abandon awareness of what you're doing. Indeed, you shouldn't *try* anything. The harder you try to relax, the more tense you'll get. That's why you may need some professional help in learning how to quiet your mind while keeping it sharply focused. Biofeedback or deep relaxation or yoga or any one of the disciplines we've mentioned may help. They sound exotic and mysterious, and may take time and patience. If you're caught meditating before a tennis game, you may also take some ribbing from your pals. But don't let that worry you. The word is getting around that fine-tuning the mind is just as important in athletics as a well-tuned body.

One thing that may help get you centered is to introduce some ritual into your game play—a set procedure to help focus your mind on the task at hand. For a swimmer, it may be showering and shaking out just so; for a runner, it could be doing warm-up exercises in the same spot every day. Using this time to get centered can help quiet your mind and focus your attention. The best pregame ritual, of course, is a long, leisurely warm-up, during which your mind is brought into play. The whole subject of warm-ups is treated in detail in Chapter 7. Here, we'll simply point out that there's a big difference between telling you to stretch your calf or "feel your calf stretching." We may say the former, but we always mean the latter. To "feel your calf stretching," you need to think about what you are doing. Find your calf in your mind's eye, focus your attention on how it feels. Is it especially tight today? As you go into your stretch, visualize what that muscle looks like, stretching, yawning, getting ready to serve. Is it feeling looser? Hotter? You should never muscle your way into a stretch by bouncing or straining or pushing, but ease into it gently, gradually nudging yourself to the edge of some discomfort but not enough to cause real pain. (This is difficult to describe but easy to feel; so don't be misled.) The best thing you could do right now, in fact, is to put this book aside and reach down to touch your toes, as you've probably done hundreds of times before. But this time, practice mind awareness. Find your zone of comfort and then edge over the boundaries of discomfort. Are your hamstrings tingling? Do your knees feel locked, or hot, or like Jell-O? While you're noting all this, be aware of your breath. Don't hold it in. Try exhaling in an exaggerated way, blowing air out through your lips, and see if that doesn't give you an extra inch or two of stretch. Come up and go down again. Shake your shoulders. Wiggle your toes. The more fun you have doing your warm-ups, the less you'll mind doing them.

When warm-ups become a daily habit, when sometimes you find yourself getting up in the middle of the day and stretching your quadriceps while using the phone, or rotating your shoulders while you wait for the elevator, then you'll know your body wisdom has taken over. And when that happens, you have also put a little more distance between yourself and the chance of getting hurt.

HOW TO BREATHE MORE FULLY AND LESSEN STRESS

(Provided by the Stress Management/ Research Program of Himalayan International Institute at Honesdale, Pennsylvania.)

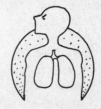

The single most important tool for control of chronic stress is the simplest and most direct—your own breathing process. Most of us breathe improperly, using only our chest muscles to force air in and out of the body. The proper and natural way of breathing is diaphragmatic breathing, utilizing the diaphragm to pull air into the lungs and to force air out again. (This is also called deep breathing, or belly breathing.) Everyone, especially athletes interested in boosting performance, should learn to breathe properly. If you breathe with only the chest muscles, expanding the chest wall, you are utilizing only about the top two-thirds of the lungs. When you breathe with the diaphragm, you are pulling air into the lower, blood-rich lobes, using all the lung capacity. The athlete who learns to breathe with the diaphragm is increasing the efficiency of the lungs by increasing the amount of oxygen/carbon dioxide exchange. This increased efficiency reduces the workload of the heart and respiratory system, resulting in decreased strain on the heart and cardiovascular system.

There are other advantages, too. Efficient, natural breathing will help you regulate your emotional and mental states and can be very useful in overcoming pain. There are several steps to master when you are increasing your awareness of, and control over, your breathing process. It takes time and practice but it is not difficult. Here is one of the exercises used by the instructors at the Himalayan Institute. It should be practiced when you are alone, at a quiet time and place, for maximum concentration and learning effectiveness.

DIAPHRAGMATIC BREATHING

The purpose of this exercise is to reestablish diaphragmatic breathing as your normal, everyday breathing process. This exercise will be most effective if you practice at least 3 times daily for 5 to 10 minutes. Eventually, the easy rhythmic motion of the diaphragmatic breathing will begin to replace the strained, habituated chest breathing. You can speed the process immeasurably by being aware of your breathing process as much as possible during the day. The more aware of your breathing pattern you become, the more often you correct the process, the faster you will replace the adverse breathing habits with the more natural and helpful diaphragmatic breathing.

To practice: Lie on your back on a rug or carpet, with a small pillow under your head. Place your left hand on your stomach, your right hand on your chest. As you breathe, concentrate on breathing into your stomach, as if you were filling your stomach with breath. Your stomach and left hand should rise with the inhalation and fall with the exhalation. The chest and right hand should not move at all. After the breath has become stable, change the rhythm of the breath to a 2:1 ratio. That is, exhale twice as long as you inhale. You are not trying to fill or empty the lungs completely, only altering the motion of the lungs. The 2:1 rhythm should be very comfortable and gentle. Simply slow the exhalation slightly and inhale slightly faster until a comfortable 2:1 rhythm is attained. (This exercise is very important. If you do only one exercise, it should be diaphragmatic breathing.)

6. Nutrition

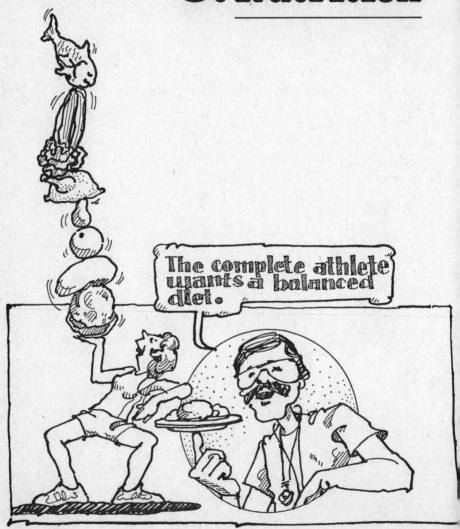

Dear Dr. Jock:

I read somewhere that you shouldn't drink water while you're exercising because it'll give you cramps. Then I read somewhere else that you should keep drinking if you exercise a lot because otherwise you risk getting dehydrated. I never get thirsty, but I am confused. Can you help.

B.L., Detroit, Michigan

Dear Dr. Jock:

My son is 15, a big, strapping sports nut who is hoping to make the starting basketball team next year. He's always had an endless amount of energy but lately I've been noticing that he poops out about 4 o'clock in the afternoon. Of all my five children, he's always been the worst eater and I'm wondering if he shouldn't start taking some vitamins or something to pep him up a little bit. What do you say?

C.K., Atlanta, Georgia

Dear Dr. Jock:

I'm in a big tennis tournament next month and I'd like to know what sorts of foods I should eat to give me extra energy. P.S. I'm allergic to spinach.

P.F., Miami, Florida

It's no wonder athletes are confused when it comes to nutrition and sports. We are all inundated with conflicting information about what to eat, when to drink and how many vitamin supplements equal a mile.

We know our meals should be "well balanced"—but does that mean weighing 4 ounces of yogurt for every 4 ounces of Cheetos? And what's wrong with junk food anyway? Frank Shorter is known to dine on hot buttered Babka and Rolaids; that top jock Reggie Jackson has lent his name to a gooey chocolate bar, and superhero Bruce Jenner goes on TV and declares Wheaties to be the Breakfast of Champions. The messages are mixed and the media are no help at all because they're always carrying pro and con stories on vitamins, additives, vegetarianism, our vast waistlines and a variety of other controversial nutritional issues that only tend to confuse us more.

The chances are that you had some sort of basic nutrition course when you were growing up. Deep down in our memories, nearly all of us can recall something important being said about the Four Basic Food Groups. Some of us can even recall feeling sorry that sausage pizza wasn't one of them.

But that was long ago, and in the meantime our minds have been swayed, our stomachs have been led to accept foods that are highly processed and vitamin depleted. But once you care about fitness, you just naturally begin to care about how foods affect your stamina, performance and endurance. You want straightforward information that will affect your running, your tennis, your general health and well-being. This chapter can help you get started.

THE BETTER YOU EAT, THE BETTER YOU PLAY

Dr. Roger Williams, the biochemist who discovered pantothenic acid, has written, "The quality of human experience, the uniquely human ability to reason, to produce art and poetry, to appreciate music or beauty, the presence of an inner life, is affected by the quality of nutrition we take into ourselves." That goes for sports performance, too. The food you eat, the vitamins and minerals you take, the chemicals, additives and preservatives you may swallow, all affect your total being. We believe that eating a nutritious mix of wholesome foods can do much to help you boost your prowess on the playing field and reduce the risk of injury.

If you've scheduled an afternoon tennis game, and just beforehand you down a thick, juicy slice of prime rib, you can expect to feel sluggish and sloppy on the court. Your blood supply will be busy helping your stomach digest the protein you've just dumped into it, and your working muscles will be deprived of their full share of nutrients. You'll be at your best if you run, swim, play tennis, cycle and so on, with a minimum of food in your stomach. Digestion takes energy; and if your body is still "out to lunch" when you want it to go to work, your game is bound to suffer. Similarly, although wolfing down two Cokes and a chocolate bar just before you start your early evening run may give you a shot of extra energy, after 5 or 10 minutes you can expect your blood sugar to drop, leaving you tired and depressed.

Knowing what and how much and when to eat and drink is important to keeping fit. The problem is that up until recently nutrition hasn't been regarded as important by most doctors. Food and diet are absolutely essential in many non-western medical systems and herbs, minerals and natural-remedy foods have been used to treat patients for thousands of years, but the vast majority of M.D.'s in this country don't know beans about nutrition. They don't even know beans *are* nutrition: they just think they're there for gas.

"The teaching of nutrition in most medical schools was, and still is miserable," says famed nutritionist Dr. Jean Mayer. It is miserable by intent. Until recently—and the change in med school curriculum is occurring, slow but steady—nutrition was simply not considered an important factor in the care and healing of sick people, especially injured athletes. If nutrition was taught at all, the class was either an electiveor poorly attended.

The reason for the Western medical establishment's benign neglect of this all-important discipline is long and complex and probably goes all the way back to the philosopher Descartes who, in helping separate our Western minds from our Western bodies, also managed to cut us off from our food supply: the "we are" from the "what we eat." Our medical schools have always preferred this less mystical, purely mechanistic view of the body. Drugs and manufactured medicines were the new desired treatments; ancient remedies, natural herb and vitamin therapies were lumped in with eye of newt, and lost. By concentrating so brilliantly on crisis intervention and relieving symptoms, most doctors have been able to get away with knowing very little about the complex and precarious links between the mind and the body and the foods that fuel them both.

Old myths and misinformation about food and its relationship to fitness are beginning to be exposed, and recreational athletes are getting the message, thanks to important research studies that are now going on. Players have always been looking for the combination of foods and artificial supplements that will boost their performance, increase their stamina and help them win. Clearly, there is no single all-round diet answering these demands. Human beings are distinct individuals with widely varying nutritional needs. Some athletes get along very well on the "recommended" 45 milligrams of vitamin C a day; others regularly take 2 grams a day, or even more if they feel a cold coming on. Most pros would laugh a team doc out of the locker room if he came round giving out cod liver oil by the spoonful, but a nutritionist named Dale Alexander says he cured Ernie Banks's bum knees and Yogi Berra's anemic batting average by prescribing doses of this natural lubricating oil (wild cherry flavor).

Nobody can say, in the present state of nutrition, just what will work and what won't. And while guidelines and recommended levels and supernutritional therapies are being worked out, it's up to each of us to be aware of what we need to make our bodies work and feel our best. If you sincerely believe that a concoction of brewer's yeast, bananas, bran flakes and lecithin helps you run farther, or putt better, or shoot more accurately from the free-throw line, then we'd be crazy to rule it out. (David still thinks that the cod liver oil is basically weird, however.)

Our point is, if you are taking the time and making the effort to eat properly, you probably don't need all the vitamins, minerals and special health food extras. At least you don't need them physiologically, though psychologically you may still find that they give you a boost.

Most nutritionists agree that as a nation we do not eat a particularly well-balanced diet. They keep telling us that the all-American diet is loaded with sugar, salt, refined flours, processed foods, saturated fats, meat protein, additives and chemical preservatives, all belonging to the category of Excessive Intake. More than 50 million Americans are considered obese, and many millions more are so much overweight that their health, not to mention their tennis games, is endangered.

The authors of *The Changing American Diet*, put out by the Center for Science in the Public Interest, surveyed changes in our eating habits between 1910 and 1976. They found that we eat many more fatty foods than we used to. Back in 1910, the average American got 32 percent of his or her daily calorie supply from fats. But now, on an average, fats supply 42 percent of our daily calories. (Remember, that's just an average. If you are a big meat-eater and can't stay away from the nuts, chocolates, butter and so on, your percentage would be even higher.) Meanwhile, the consumption of complex carbohydrates has dropped considerably, which is too bad because complex carbohydrates—slow-burning starches—fuel our bodies most efficiently.

As you'd expect, the nationwide consumption of refined sugars rose 50 percent, from 12 to 18 percent of our total intake; for the average American, this breaks down to somewhere between 90 and 170 pounds of sugar a year. Protein intake has remained fairly constant throughout the 66-year period. Many of us eat two or three times more protein than we need—the kind of overload that can give an athlete real problems.

HOW CAN TOO MUCH PROTEIN BE A PROBLEM? AREN'T ATHLETES SUPPOSED TO LOAD UP ON PROTEIN?

It is time to destroy Nutrition Myth Number 1. For as long as you can remember, you've probably heard your teachers, trainers, doctors, mates, mothers and fellow jocks preaching the value of a lot of protein. If a little red meat is good for you, a juicy 16-ounce porterhouse just before a big game must be better. Massive advertising has helped make high protein synonymous with high performance, strength, energy and winning. The stereotypical training table for jocks was laden with thick steaks, butter and cheeses; in many unfortunate cases, it still is. Now we know this regimen was a big mistake. Protein is a vital nutrient and absolutely essential when it comes to building strong muscles and healthy bones. But protein is not the key to high energy. Carbohydrates are. Protein, it turns out, is the least efficient energy source. It can actually sap your strength, because it requires so much energy and oxygen to break down its large, complex molecules into usable sugar. More important, protein metabolism demands so much body water to flush out the waste products, ammonia and urea, that it opens up the very real danger of dehydration. (If the waste products are *not* flushed out, they can build up and cause you to feel exhausted and washed out.) We know now that your body runs best and most efficiently on the glucose that it gets from a wide variety of sugars and starches. Naturally, it gets more usable energy from some carbohydrates than others. Don't think that a steady diet of M&M's, Twinkies and Kool-Aid will keep you in shape. Not only is too much sugar frowned on because of its links to elevated blood triglycerides and cholesterol, the fact is that gobbling up candy, pastries, ice cream, soda pop and even those special sugary athletic drinks within an hour before an endurance event can actually depress your ability to perform. This is because the sugar stimulates the pancreas, and out pours the insulin. Then, before the athlete knows what hit him, there is a sudden drop in blood glucose. In performance terms, the muscles are robbed of essential nutrients, concentration is disrupted and the body is not getting the nourishment it needs. You will function better if you take time to pace your eating: small amounts of carbohydrates at regular intervals—especially raw fruits and fresh vegetables. It's interesting to note that sugar snacks affect the body differently once it is exercising, which is why we recommend taking mildly sugared fluids at regular intervals during a long endurance event, to help keep the glucose supply up. You can get the supply of carbohydrates you need from a wide range of foods, including fresh fruit, bread, spaghetti, waffles, pancakes, corn, rice, potatoes, beans and all sorts of vegetables.

The old steak-and-scrambled-eggs meal before the Big Game must now give way to a well-balanced diet—one high in carbohydrates, moderate in fat and relatively low in protein. The American Heart Association recommends a balance of 35 percent fats, 51 percent carbohydrates, and 14 percent protein, and that sounds right to us.

DOESN'T EATING A LOT OF RED MEAT HELP REPLENISH MUSCLES?

That used to be the thinking—all the way back to the Greeks, who ate bull meat so they would be strong as a bull. Well, it's bull all right. In fact, if you're careful about balancing proteins, and getting adequate supplies of vitamin B12, you can do very nicely without eating meat at all. In general, we recommend that you limit the amount of animal protein you eat. Meats, cheese and eggs tend to be high in saturated fat; and people with high levels of saturated fat in their diet are much more susceptible to heart disease, stroke and some forms of cancer. Instead, we recommend that you eat more fish and chicken, more fruits and vegetables, more beans and bran and whole grains, and try to keep red meat down to no more than three or four servings—or less—a week.

We notice that as people work themselves into shape, they naturally tend to eat less meat. Some find it too heavy, too filling and—according to how high their health consciousness has been raised—too overloaded with food coloring, pesticides, herbicides, antibiotics and other suspect substances. Eating a lot of red meat (and processed foods) these days involves too many dangers and unknowns.

WHY IS WATER SO IMPORTANT? HOW MUCH SHOULD WE DRINK?

Water is the single most important nutrient in the human body. You can get along for a good long while without food, but if the body is deprived of water for even a few days, the metabolic machinery shuts down, the delicate sodium-potassium balance is upset, and it dies.

The more active you are, the more water you lose through sweat and panting, and the more of it you need to keep your body from overheating and to flush out by-products of cell metabolism. How much water is enough depends on your size, your condition, the heat of the day and the energy cost of what you're doing. To avoid heat injuries, everyone ought to start off with about two glasses before playing. A conditioned badminton player who burns up about 350 calories in an hour on a cool overcast day will require less water replacement than an overweight novice on a bicycle, sweating out a 13-mile run at 660 calories per hour. Professional athletes may actually weigh in before and after a game or practice to assess exactly how much fluid they've lost. The pros figure that for every pound of weight lost, they should consume at least a pint of fluid. When you lose body water—even as little as 3 percent of the total—your performance is really diminished. And dehydration can be the underlying cause of all sorts of sports mishaps. Lack of water can throw your whole game off, and make you feel dizzy, nauseous, weak and uncomfortable. If you ignore the symptoms and your body continues to overheat, you can collapse and die. Too often, players don't even know the problem is dehydration because they associate their need for water with a feeling of thirst. If you wait to get thirsty you are already behind in your water requirements. When you're out there, being active, using energy, you shouldn't wait to feel thirsty. You should drink freely, but not overload your system with a half-gallon gulp. If you're getting ready for an endurance event, a good tip is to drink until you have to pee. Then you know you're hydrated. While you play, you're better off drinking small amounts at frequent intervals. Runners who do from 8 to 10 miles or more should drink plenty before they run, and shouldn't resist stopping if there's a convenient drinking fountain along the way. Water is especially crucial to long-distance runners, cross-country skiers and other athletes whose sports require a maximum of energy over long periods of time.

WHAT ABOUT THOSE SPECIAL SPORTS DRINKS?

Nutrition Myth Number 2 bites the dust. Those special high-energy, thirst-quenching, electrolyte-balancing drinks that are supposed to replenish body fluids have not proved any better for you than good clean American water. They may taste better, and give you a great boost psychologically, but physiologically you are probably just as well off replacing water with water. Sometimes, if your workout has been particularly strenuous, you might benefit from a pinch of salt in the water (1 teaspoon to 6 quarts should be enough to prevent heat exhaustion). And very small quantities of potassium could be necessary if your diet isn't adequate, or if you are taking a diuretic. If you want a little sweetness, add fresh lemon juice or some other fruit juice. But don't confuse good nutrition with a good advertising campaign.

WHAT ABOUT SALT TABLETS AND ANABOLIC STEROIDS?

We've lumped these two together because they are both remedies that athletes take—and shouldn't. Indeed, both can be dangerous and should be avoided. If you're drinking enough fluid, salt tablets should be unnecessary. Most likely, you are getting all the salt you need now in your diet, and if you're a typical American you're probably getting far too much of it, sneakily added by food manufacturers to all sorts of canned, processed and packaged goods. Too much salt in the diet is related to hypertension and stroke, and it should be avoided because it throws off the delicate balance of the body fluids that bathe the cells and keep them active. Too much salt concentrated outside body cells leaches out precious intracellular fluid. This imbalance can be a real problem when you're doing vigorous exercise and counting on all the intracellular machinery to help you produce energy. Remember: you need water when you exercise, not additional salt.

Anabolic steroids are a different story, and much more dangerous. For a while, steroids were popular among athletes—primarily professional ones—because they were supposed to increase strength and improve performance. They seemed to work for certain members of the East European teams in the Olympics, and they have—or had—quite a following in the United States. But now steroids have been shown to have many more minuses than pluses, and we recommend that athletes stay away from them altogether. They can cause premature closure of growth centers in children, liver damage, skin problems, testicular atrophy and, in women, hirsutism (excessive hair), male-pattern baldness and alterations in the menstrual cycle. Several studies have shown that steroids and a regular strength program are no more efficient than the strength program alone.

ARE VITAMIN AND MINERAL SUPPLEMENTS IN THE SAME CATEGORY WITH SALT TABLETS AND STEROIDS?

Absolutely not. We know that salt tablets and steroids can be dangerous; we are only beginning to understand the value of vitamins and mineral supplements, especially as they apply to both the prevention and the treatment of sports injuries. This is a complex and controversial issue. For the time being, the consensus seems to be that if you are eating a proper diet and getting adequate amounts of nutrients from the four basic food groups (milk and milk products, meat and high-protein foods, fruits and vegetables, cereal and grain foods) plus plenty of bran, you most likely have no need for extra vitamin or mineral supplements.

The crucial consideration here is, ". . . *if* you are eating a proper diet and getting adequate amounts of nutrients. . . ." How do we know if we are eating a proper diet, let alone what a proper diet consists of? Do you, for example, have any idea what the percentage breakdown is of fats, carbohydrates and proteins in your own present food intake? (That's why the recommendation of the American Heart Association, and ourselves, that you eat 35 percent fats, 51 percent carbohydrates and 14 percent protein, is less useful than it might be.) How much protein is there in a serving of liver? A slice of cheese? A sliver of pecan pie? Can you name all the carbohydrates you ate today? Can you name ten high-fat foods that should be avoided? Can you name five of those that you haven't eaten in the last two days? And what about your sugar intake? If you're smart, you've been cutting down. Do you realize how much sugar you take in without even knowing it's there? Did you know that one 8-ounce bottle of soda pop has about 5 teaspoons of granulated sugar in it, that 1 tablespoon of jelly may have the equivalent of 6 teaspoons of sugar and 4 ounces of hard candy the equivalent of about 20? And what about vitamins and minerals? How much vitamin A, B_6 and B_{12}, C, D and E are you getting now? How much do you need?

All of which brings us to another problem that compounds our ignorance and makes us even more confused—the so-called nutrition experts can't seem to agree on what constitutes an adequate level of nutrients, especially when it comes to vitamins and minerals. More and more, we hear talk about the difference between the minimal requirement of a vitamin to avoid telling signs of deficiency and the amount desirable for *optimal* health and performance. Nutritionists certainly know how much B1 (thiamin) and vitamin C we all need to prevent beriberi and scurvy, but what is really the relation between vitamin C and colds? Or between vitamin E and healing? Who is to say that 15 units of vitamin E is "adequate" if, in fact, an extra 50 can be easily tolerated by the body and will clear up those leg cramps you've been getting after you run?

There are questions that won't be answered here, but that will be answered someday, and you should be paying attention. If you're at all typical, and are still getting 60 or 70 percent of your nutrients from fats and sugars, then maybe something *is* missing from your diet. You may not be making yourself sick, but you may be falling far short of optimal wellness if you're not fueling your body with the most efficient, beneficial foods. We can't be sure, and neither can you until you make a point of developing some real nutritional awareness. We don't want to encourage you to spend your money on spurious or superfluous remedies, but we'd be foolish not to recognize the value some athletes seem to find in this magic powder, or that capsule, or those extra vitamins. If a tennis player chooses to believe that his "energy shake" of safflower oil, lecithin and powdered yeast makes him a stronger, faster, more formidable competitor, who can say that that extra edge of confidence won't really help his game? As long as you're careful not to overdo it with the fat-soluble vitamins A-D-E-K (they're stored in the liver, and if the levels there get too high, you could develop toxic side effects), and as long as you realize that you *may* be wasting your money, you won't be doing yourself any harm. You may, in fact, be helping—but it's really up to you.

As research continues, and the needs of athletes under stress become clearer, we will undoubtedly see more nutrition-related therapies. Some will work and some won't—only time and careful research will tell which. In the meantime, we're at a hit-or-miss, trial-and-error stage. Certainly there's hardly a trainer around who won't admit to passing off some vitamin C to his players every now and then, especially when one of them feels a cold coming up. And both C and vitamin B complex are gaining a reputation among athletes concerned about reducing stress and battling the effects of pollution on their air-gulping bodies. Vitamin E is another oft-touted remedy for a variety of medical complaints. Believers have long been asserting that it boosts their energy and increases their endurance, sexual and otherwise. Increasing numbers of researchers including Dr. Roy

Bruder, psychobiologist, say that urban athletes need higher-than-usual doses of vitamin E to help them in their constant struggle against nitrous oxide, ozone and car engine exhaust.

Another sports-related use for vitamin E comes from its reputation as a helpful aid in easing circulation. Some athletes who tend to get leg cramps at night are finding relief from relatively high doses of vitamin E, up to 1,000 units daily.

Many women athletes who are iron deficient (and many women are, especially if they use an IUD and have heavy menstrual flow) find that iron supplements really have a positive effect on performance. It may also be that people who are deficient in magnesium are more prone to sudden heart attack during exercise. This usually unchecked mineral seems to be important in preventing the cardiac arrhythmia that causes athletes with no history of heart disease whatsoever to drop dead on the tennis court or golf course. To prevent such an occurrence, some patients with a magnesium deficiency take dolomite tablets, which contain high levels of magnesium. Actually, some runners have long insisted that magnesium—taken either in tablet form or naturally, in fruits, whole grains, brown rice, fresh beans and peas—helps prevent leg cramps.

Since it is so tricky to set nutritional guidelines to fit everyone, we suggest that you spend a little time studying and evaluating your own eating plan. Develop an awareness of what foods you currently eat and how they affect your performance. Does an iron supplement for borderline anemia turn into a winning burst of energy on the racquetball court? Is your 12-mile run made any more pleasant by drinking three glasses of water before you begin? Try writing down every single thing—every potato chip, every buttered half bagel, every sliver of pie—that you eat for two weeks, and then see what a nutritionist has to say about your eating regimen. (Some doctors who practice nutrition-related therapies ask for a hair sample, too, to be used in a complete mineral analysis.) But resist falling prey to all the hullabaloo about Instant Energy anything. Contrary to the popular misconception, vitamins do not give you energy. Foods give you energy; what vitamins do—or so it is thought—is to regulate the metabolic process.

WHAT IS CARBOHYDRATE LOADING?

This is a high-performance eating regimen developed by a team of Swedish physiologists. It is based on the idea that the more glycogen you can pack into muscle tissue just before performing in an endurance sport such as running, distance swimming or cross-country skiing, the more energy you'll have to call on to keep up your performance and stamina. It's not for everyone, though. Increasing numbers of athletes are going in for carbohydrate loading, especially marathoners. They report that the legendary wall of agony you hit at 20 miles—when your body is out of fuel and running up a painful oxygen debt—is more easily run through after careful carbohydrate loading. The plan sounds deceptively simple. An athlete first begins to exhaust glycogen stored in the muscles by taking a long run—maybe for about 90 minutes. This is combined with a 3-day diet limited to fats and proteins—meat, fish, eggs and cheese. Carbohydrates are either eliminated completely or kept to a maximum of 100 grams. During this time, the marathon runner continues to train. However, with all the glycogen gone from his system, he is likely to feel tired and out of sorts. During the last three days before the race, the runner stops training and loads up his diet with foods high in carbohydrate and low in salt and residue. The Swedish team showed that glycogen levels could almost be tripled through this regimen.

But even though carbohydrate loading can be useful for some serious athletes willing to go through with it, it may not be useful or even healthy for everyone. Some bodies just can't take it. You'll have to listen to yours to find out. Some runners get sick from it, or feel they actually tire more quickly in the race than if they hadn't loaded up on carbohydrates at all. Certainly it's geared to endurance sports such as running and cross-country skiing and never intended for tennis or basketball players. If you want to experiment with it, take it by slow, easy degrees, and don't force yourself beyond your limits. And in any event, you shouldn't do it more than 2 or 3 times a year.

WHAT ABOUT COFFEE?

Coffee used to be on the list of no-no's before a competition. The thinking was that too much caffeine increased urine production and decreased the body's water supply. But there is new evidence to suggest that a cup of double-strength coffee drunk an hour before an endurance contest might be very helpful to the athlete who is looking for ways to tap an alternative energy supply: fat. It seems that caffeine, by stimulating the sympathetic nervous system, causes the cells to release free fatty acids. This assures the long-distance athlete of a bigger energy supply and thus—all other things being equal—of an improved performance. This preliminary conclusion was reported by Dr. David Costill, director of the Human Performance Laboratory at Ball State University, Muncie, Indiana, one of the leading authorities on exercise physiology. It doesn't work for everyone, he cautions—but as you must have realized by now, nothing in nutrition does.

WILL EXERCISE HELP IN LOSING WEIGHT?

This is not a diet book. But we can answer this often-asked question with an emphatic, unequivocal Yes. Exercise can be a wonderful aid in losing weight, and we'd be suspicious of any diet plan that didn't involve you in some sort of regular workout. Anything that gets you moving is better than sitting around counting calories until the next feeding. The trick to losing weight is no trick at all. It is simply that you have to expend more calories than you consume. If you burn up about the same number as you take in, your weight will remain the same. If you burn up less, you'll gain . . . and gain . . . and go on gaining until you finally decide to do something about it. One of the smartest things you can do is to get hooked on exercise. In addition to the number of calories it burns up every minute, regular exercise can actually act as a natural appetite suppressant. True, if you do no more than walk two blocks or bowl a single game, when you stop you may still feel that uncontrollable urge to replenish the energy you've spent with something sinful from Sara Lee. But if you stick to a conditioning program, and begin cutting things out of your normal eating pattern, you will most assuredly lose weight. How much will depend on what you have to lose and what you do to lose it.

To lose one pound of body fat, you have to expend about 3,500 more calories than you consume. Different sports use up varying numbers of calories. Running at about 10 miles an hour for one hour will burn up 900 calories; bicycling a leisurely 5½ mph will burn up only 210 in an hour. If you do 30 minutes of brisk walking every day (burning up 5.2 calories per minute) and meanwhile eat 400 calories less each day than you've been doing, it will take 27 days to lose 5 pounds. If you double your walking time and knock 800 calories off your daily intake, after about 26 days you will have lost 10 pounds. We've included some charts at the end of this chapter that can be helpful if you're serious about exercising to lose weight. In a little book called *Exercise Equivalents of Foods* (Southern Illinois University Press, Carbondale, $1.95), Frank Konishi runs through a long list of common foods and tells you how much exercise you need to work that food off. For instance, a hot dog with ketchup (258 calories) can be exercised off by 31 minutes of swimming or 26 minutes of jogging. You can work off a 50-calorie chocolate-chip cookie with a 10-minute walk or an 8-minute bike ride, but a jelly donut at 226 calories will cost you 27 minutes of swimming or a 44-minute walk just to stay even.

SOME FINAL CAUTIONS ON NUTRITION

Your local health food store may offer a nice variety of wholesome natural foods, but so can the supermarket, if you stick to the dairy case, and the fresh-fruits-and-vegetable, fish-and-poultry and whole-grain aisles.

Whether you're deciding on a pregame meal or a complete change in your present eating habits, be sure to choose foods that you like, that agree with you and that don't leave you feeling stuffed or uncomfortable. Learn to listen to and trust your own digestive system. Stan the Marathon Man may wolf down a huge pancake breakfast soaked in maple syrup a few hours before a big run, but that doesn't mean it's best for you. Some athletes prefer to eat nothing before a meet. You'll need to experiment and discover which foods best suit you and your life-style. Don't force yourself to follow someone else's eating plan, and if there are certain foods that you feel you must have to make yourself a champion, include them!

For optimal ease and performance, it's probably best not to start really vigorous physical exercise until three or four hours after a meal. The idea, basically, is to have as little as possible in the stomach so that all your energy is directed to the activity. A wait of one or two hours is acceptable, since probably there will be enough glycogen already stored in the liver and muscles to see you comfortably through a 10-mile run or an hour of tennis. Wrestlers, gymnasts, rowers and others in sports that put the abdominal muscles through the ringer should not eat immediately before working out. Swimmers shouldn't either, because—just as your mother told you—you really can get cramps if you've recently loaded up on a heavy meal.

Don't get so hung up on the complexities of proper nutrition that it takes all the fun out of eating, training or playing. The more you exercise, the better your condition will be, and the more inclined you'll be to eat sensibly. Let the changes happen naturally. If you've been a meat-and-white-bread man all your life, don't think you have to switch to tofu cakes and alfalfa sprouts overnight. It takes time to develop fitness and it takes time to develop the body wisdom that will lead to the best diet for you.

ENERGY EQUIVALENTS OF FOOD

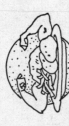

MINUTES REQUIRED TO BURN UP CALORIES

Average serving	Calories	Running 10 mph 900 cal/h	Cycling 13 mph 660 cal/h	Jogging 5 mph 500 cal/h	Swimming 1/4 mph 300 cal/h	Walking 2½ mph 200 cal/h
Bacon (3 strips)	175	12	16	21	35	53
Corned beef	225	15	21	27	45	68
Rib roast (medium)	340	23	31	41	68	102
Steak	235	15	21	27	45	68
Hot dog	140	10	14	18	30	45
Ham	400	27	36	48	80	120
Pork sausage	180	12	16	21	35	53
Fried chicken (thigh and leg)	330	22	31	40	68	101
Fried fish	210	14	18	25	41	61
Hamburger	390	20	35	47	80	120
Cheese sandwich	325	22	30	39	65	97
Peanut butter sandwich	365	24	33	44	73	109
Vegetable soup	90	7	9	11	19	29
Corn (1 ear)	100	7	9	12	20	30
Potato, mashed	100	7	9	12	20	30
Blue cheese dressing	150	10	14	18	30	45

MINUTES REQUIRED TO BURN UP CALORIES

Average serving	Calories	Running 10 mph 900 cal/h	Cycling 13 mph 660 cal/h	Jogging 5 mph 500 cal/h	Swimming 1/4 mph 300 cal/h	Walking 2½ mph 200 cal/h
Butter (1 tbsp.)	110	7	9	12	21	31
Mayonnaise (2 tbsp.)	220	15	20	27	45	68
Vegetable oil (2 tbsp.)	270	18	23	31	51	76
Biscuits (2)	100	7	9	12	20	30
Cornbread	200	14	18	24	40	60
Cheese cake	300	20	27	36	60	90
Chocolate cake	400	27	36	48	80	120
Chocolate ice cream	250	18	23	30	50	75
Mince pie	500	35	45	60	100	150
Strawberry shortcake	300	20	27	36	60	90
Candy bar	450	30	40	54	90	135
Malted milk	450	30	40	54	90	135
Cocoa	120	8	10	13	21	31
Milk	165	11	15	20	35	52
Beer (8 oz.)	115	8	10	13	21	31

DAYS REQUIRED TO LOSE 5 TO 25 POUNDS
BY SWIMMING* AND LOWERING DAILY CALORIE INTAKE

Minutes of swimming	Reduction of calories per day (in kcal)	Days to lose 5 lbs.	Days to lose 10 lbs.	Days to lose 15 lbs.	Days to lose 20 lbs.	Days to lose 25 lbs.
30	400	23	46	69	92	115
30	600	18	36	52	72	90
30	800	14	28	42	56	70
30	1,000	12	24	36	48	60
45	400	19	38	57	76	95
45	600	15	30	45	60	75
45	800	13	26	39	52	65
45	1,000	11	22	33	44	55
60	400	16	32	48	64	80
60	600	14	28	42	56	70
60	800	11	22	33	44	55
60	1,000	10	20	30	40	50

*Swimming at about 30 yards/minute calculated at 8.5 cal/minute. Reproduced from *Exercise Equivalents of Foods* by Frank Konishi (copyright © 1973, Southern Illinois University Press).

DAYS REQUIRED TO LOSE 5 TO 25 POUNDS BY JOGGING* AND LOWERING DAILY CALORIE INTAKE

Minutes of jogging	Reduction of calories per day (in kcal)	Days to lose 5 lbs.	Days to lose 10 lbs.	Days to lose 15 lbs.	Days to lose 20 lbs.	Days to lose 25 lbs.
30	400	21	42	63	84	105
30	600	17	34	51	68	85
30	800	14	28	42	58	70
30	1,000	12	24	36	48	60
45	400	18	36	54	72	90
45	600	14	28	42	56	70
45	800	12	24	36	48	60
45	1,000	10	20	30	40	50
60	400	15	30	45	60	75
60	600	12	24	36	48	60
60	800	11	22	33	44	55
60	1,000	9	18	27	36	45

*Jogging—calculated at 10 cal/minute. Reproduced from *Exercise Equivalents of Foods* by Frank Konishi (copyright © 1973, Southern Illinois University Press).

DAYS REQUIRED TO LOSE 5 TO 25 POUNDS
BY BICYCLING* AND LOWERING DAILY CALORIE INTAKE

Minutes of bicycling	Reduction of calories per day (in kcal)	Days to lose 5 lbs.	Days to lose 10 lbs.	Days to lose 15 lbs.	Days to lose 20 lbs.	Days to lose 25 lbs.
30	400	25	50	75	100	125
30	600	19	38	57	76	95
30	800	17	34	51	68	85
30	1,000	13	26	39	52	65
45	400	22	44	66	88	110
45	600	17	34	51	68	85
45	800	14	28	42	56	70
45	1,000	12	24	36	48	60
60	400	19	38	57	76	95
60	600	15	30	45	60	75
60	800	13	26	39	52	65
60	1,000	11	22	33	44	55

*Bicycling calculated at 6.5 cal/minute at approximately 7 mph. Reproduced from *Exercise Equivalents of Foods* by Frank Konishi (copyright © 1973, Southern Illinois University Press).

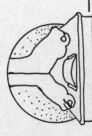

DAYS REQUIRED TO LOSE 5 TO 25 POUNDS
BY WALKING* AND LOWERING DAILY CALORIE INTAKE

Minutes of walking	Reduction of calories per day (in kcal)	Days to lose 5 lbs.	Days to lose 10 lbs.	Days to lose 15 lbs.	Days to lose 20 lbs.	Days to lose 25 lbs.
30	400	27	54	81	108	135
30	600	20	40	60	80	100
30	800	16	32	48	64	80
30	1,000	13	26	39	52	65
45	400	23	46	69	92	115
45	600	18	36	54	72	90
45	800	14	28	42	56	70
45	1,000	12	24	36	48	60
60	400	21	42	63	84	105
60	600	16	32	48	64	80
60	800	13	26	39	52	65
60	1,000	11	22	33	44	55

*Walking briskly (3.5–4.0 mph), calculated at 5.2 cal/minute. Reproduced from *Exercise Equivalents of Foods* by Frank Konishi (copyright © 1973, Southern Illinois University Press).

7. Warm-Ups

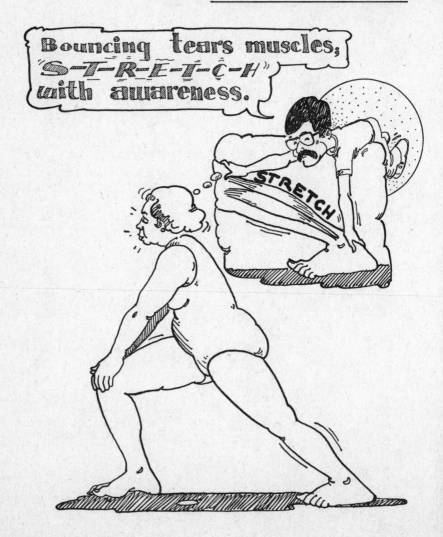

Dear Dr. Jock:

Can you please tell me the best warm-up for a runner? I'm a grandmother, 59 years old, 5'2", 103 pounds and I've been running for 4 glorious months. I started out real, real slow and now run 4 miles, 3 times a week. But I don't think I'm warming up right because I see some other runners doing things that I don't do. What is the best way?

I.L., Boston, Massachusetts

Dear Dr. Jock:

I tried cross-country skiing for my first time last year (the whole family did it—all nine of us!) and we all liked it a lot, but toward the end of the season I was getting a lot of soreness in the back of my leg, around the calf muscles. I'm worried I might really hurt them seriously this year. Any advice?

J.F., Cleveland, Ohio

Dear Dr. Jock:

I'm not very flexible and as a result, when I exercise, I tend to pull a lot of muscles. What can I do to increase my flexibility? And maybe you can tell me why it is that tight muscles hurt more than loose muscles. Is there such a thing as too loose muscles? It's not important, but I was just wondering.

W.R., Fresno, California

Every week, Dr. Jock gets letters, hundreds and hundreds of letters from runners, tennis players, skiers, hikers, weight lifters, cyclists, walkers and assorted others in this country who are involved in some sort of regular exercise routine, or want to be.

They write, not out of friendship, but out of pain. They hurt, most of them; they have some aches, pain or injury that is getting in the way of them and their good time.

99

"I was playing tennis and all of a sudden I felt a sharp pain in my calf, as though someone had crept up on the court and smashed me with their racquet . . . It hurts so much I can't bear the thought of playing tennis again. What can I do?" or . . . "I want to start running again but last time I tried my feet started to hurt me real bad and I had to quit" or . . . "I've started a swimming program for myself at my local Y and I love it except that I am getting a very sharp pain in my shoulder every time I try and lift my arms."

Though the letters are all different, and the injuries quite distinct, the underlying problem is the same—most people don't take the time they should to warm up. They know they *should*, but they don't and our telling them they should is so much water off a swimmer's back until—UNTIL—something happens. Something bad, some sign of pain or discomfort that they can't shake off.

Up until then, you and every other athlete in the world believe that sports injuries are what happens to the other guy. But when it happens to you—when your elbow feels so raw you have to cancel Tuesday's tennis game or when your running program gets cancelled on account of pain—then warm-ups take on a whole new significance.

It's unfortunately true that until you experience the need for them, warm-ups are just another something extra you don't have time for. Once you realize that you could probably eliminate 60 percent of your aches and pains and sports injuries with a simple 10-minute stretching routine, it's quite another story.

Take the story, for instance, of a runner from Phoenix, Arizona, who wrote us to share a frustrating experience that millions of athletes will understand all too well.

> During the summer of 1976 I decided to run a marathon, the Fiesta Bowl in December, 1976. Previous to this I had run about a half dozen distance races, varying from 8 to 13 miles in length. I followed a training program that I felt was realistic for a 35-year-old family man whose job demands a good deal of overtime. The eight weeks prior I averaged 40 miles a week, with a 17-miler three weeks prior to the race and a 20-miler two weeks prior. When the gun went off, I was 6'1" and 182 lbs. and I felt pretty decent. I ran the race in 3:00:54 and was completely decimated at the end.
>
> The next evening I tried to jog to loosen up, and had a very painful sensation in my right knee. I tried to run at different times for several weeks but the pain under the kneecap would not let me. I went to a doctor who injected my knee with cortisone and gave me butazoline, both of which did no good whatsoever. He finally diagnosed the problem as chondromalacia. I then went to a podiatrist who casted my feet for orthotics, which I wore, and continue to wear, in my shoes with no positive results.
>
> Finally I went to an orthopedic surgeon, who felt a surgical procedure

called a retinacular release may help my problem. Quite simply, as I understand this, by severing the ligaments on the right side of the knee it allows the patella to track differently on the femur and hopefully relieve the problem. He did this in April, 1977.

I got no relief whatsoever for several months, and finally in September, 1977, I started to jog again. No basketball, tennis, sprinting, etc., but the knee could handle a jog. I built up until in December I could run a 10K in about 40 minutes. Then in January, 1978, I ran a half marathon in about 1:31, which was a comfortable pace. However, two days later I tried to jog again and my knee was in the same shape as after the marathon. My orthopedic surgeon said he didn't know what to do, and so I went to another orthopedic surgeon a friend recommended, who had a good rep as a knee man. After looking at my old X-rays, arthrogram, surgical notes of the first doctor and analyzing a strength test of my knee, he came to the same conclusion—chondromalacia. He wanted to do an arthroscopy, and if he saw what he anticipated seeing he would shave and drill the kneecap. I have no doubt that this is what would have happened had I consented to the arthroscopy. He said I would be laid up for months and eventually work up to jogging 2 miles. This wasn't exactly what I had in mind.

By the way, during the operation the surgeon looked at the underside of the kneecap and he said it looked healthy except for two or three striations. He did have me doing straight-leg leg-lifts to build up my quadriceps also.

Well, after doctor No. 2 I was real low, but heard of another young orthopod who had worked on a lot of knees and went to see him. I will not tell you all his comments but after about an hour of going over both my knees he said that in his opinion my problem was the result of two things: (1) very tight hamstrings that I would have to stretch out and (2) a quadriceps muscle that was atrophying. The hams were tight, quite frankly, because I never had stretched before this. He told me quite simply to throw my leg up on a desk, chair, fender, etc., several times a day and do a hurdler's stretch, trying to put my chin on my knee. The quads were atrophying due to pain from the operation and lack of use and he got me back on straight-leg leg-raises.

Well, about four weeks after starting this program I was jogging again and recently ran 6 miles in 37:21, which is really quite good for me. I doubt that I will ever run a marathon again, and my knee is still weak and probably not more than 75 to 80 percent. However, with a little warm-up and a little stretching I can run again and for this I thank the Lord.

TIGHT MUSCLES TEAR; LOOSE MUSCLES STRETCH

The fact is that the older we get, the tighter we get. And tight muscles can tear when they're subjected to the kind of stress and stretch they naturally get in sports. Muscles that are not warmed up transmit more force to the tendons they're attached to. And continued pulling on the tendons can cause microscopic tears, the precursor to that common sports ailment known as tendinitis. Since tendons receive a sparse supply of blood, when one has been injured it heals slowly. That's why a severe tennis elbow or damage to an Achilles tendon may keep you from fully enjoying your sport for more than a year.

We're assuming you're finally convinced that a tight muscle is more easily hurt than a flexible muscle, and that the best way to loosen it is by continued gentle stretching. Now you'll need a plan, a stretching routine that you'll do every day. Advice on proper warm-ups is woven all through this book. In this chapter we're concerned with the nuts and bolts of body-stretching: which stretch works for each major part of the body.

First, though, a couple of cautions.

If you're not paying attention to what you're doing, even a 20-minute stretch may leave you cold. Your mind has got to be involved. When your body is really responding, 10 minutes a day should be enough. Naturally, if you do more, you'll benefit more.

Second, just as critical as warming up your muscles before you use them is cooling them down *after* you've exercised. That's because as you exercise, your body is breaking down muscle tissue. When you're through working hard, if you don't ease off and flush the pooled blood and breakdown products from your system, they can build up in your muscles. The result may be pain and cramps later on. So, when you're through running or playing tennis or whatever, don't stop and sit down all at once. Take 5 or 10 minutes to walk around slowly and stretch. After you work out is an especially good time to stretch because then the muscles are warm and loose. This slight squeezing action is what you need to keep the blood flowing and the late-night leg cramps away.

TIPS FOR STRETCHING

KEEP IT SLOW AND RHYTHMIC

Many of our best stretches come to us from yoga, along with the very good advice that stretches should be done slowly and rhythmically. Listen for your own body's natural, flowing beat. Don't jerk, don't bounce and don't forget about your breathing. When you feel a good stretch, hold it, relax, exhale and see how easy it becomes to stretch a little further. Again, the yoga masters teach the importance of breath awareness and control if you're keen on stretching your body to its fullest.

SET YOUR OWN PACE

Although we recommend the number of times each stretch should be done, you needn't hold to it if it's uncomfortable. It's better to do the stretch fewer times and build up slowly than to push yourself too hard. If your stretching routine is painful, you won't want to do it. Accept the fact that on some days you may stretch a little less and on some days more—and one day it'll be as much a part of your daily routine as washing your face or combing your hair.

KNOW WHAT YOU'RE DOING

Read over the exercise thoroughly before you try it. Get a good sense of what it is you're supposed to do. Conjure up a mental image of yourself actually doing it. The more ways you can think of to bring your mind into play while you stretch your body, the better off you'll be.

MAKE IT A RITUAL

Begin each session, if at all possible, with a few minutes of deep breathing and total relaxation. If you don't know how to do that, study the diaphragmatic breathing exercise at the end of Chapter 5. Try to do your stretching routine in the same place, at approximately the same time. Don't just plop down in the den, with the coffeetable closing in on one side and your 11-year-old on the other asking what's for dinner. Set aside a time and a space if you possibly can. On the other hand, there's nothing wrong with sneaking in a stretch on the run—at the office, waiting for an elevator, standing in line at the checkout counter. It may look a little strange, but so does wearing a neck brace.

WORK ON BODY AWARENESS

There are several systems around for increasing your ability to stretch—yoga, Feldenkreis, the Alexander technique, bioenergetics. A technique we especially like is a combination of contracting and relaxing your muscles, based in part on Jacobson's pioneering work in Progressive Relaxation. To help people become more aware of what relaxed, stretched muscles feel like he has them experience the opposite—tense, hard muscles. (Sensing the difference may take some time, but it will develop as your body awareness increases. You can read more about Progressive Relaxation in Chapter 2 of Barbara Brown's classic in the body-mind field, *Stress and the Art of Biofeedback*.) So, to put a little more educated stretch in a muscle, first contract it as tightly as you can. When you let go it automatically retreats to a more relaxed state. That's the feeling you want to develop. You can use the same principle in toe touching. Bend over and try to reach down to your toes, keeping your knees straight. Then squat down for 5 seconds. Then repeat the toe touch. You'll find you've picked up a few inches.

Another seeing-is-believing stretch involves sitting with your back against a wall and spreading your legs as far apart as possible. Have someone mark the distance. Then bring your feet together and squeeze them as hard as you can—an isometric contraction. Spread them open again and see how much more stretch you get this time.

PUTTING TOGETHER YOUR OWN WARM-UP PROGRAM

The best warm-up program is the one you put together for yourself, based on solid information and sound medical advice. The charts below spell out everything you need to know. Find your sport, note the major muscle groups you need to work on and go through the list of possible exercises to see which suit you best. In each of the categories—quadriceps, hamstrings, calves and so on—we've tried to give you a few choices. Try one for a while, and vary the exercises from time to time so that your warm-up routine won't get too stale or boring. You can't afford to let it get boring. It's too important.

WHAT'S THE BEST WARM-UP?

For each sport we've indicated with an X the body parts that must be stretched prior to play. Feel free to supplement with other stretches too; the more flexible you are, the safer you'll be. Specific exercises follow. Remember: warm-ups are a major factor in preventing sports injuries. Try to do them every day.

STRETCHING THE CALF

Tight calves are a leading cause of injury in a wide variety of sports. Women especially have to pay attention to this muscle area because years of wearing high heels has left many women with extremely short, contracted calf muscles.

	Calf	Hamstrings	Quadriceps
Running	X	X	X
Swimming			
Cycling	X	X	X
Skiing	X	X	X
Racquet sports	X	X	
Golf			
Bat and ball	X	X	
Basketball, volleyball	X	X	X
Soccer, football	X	X	X

THE WALL LEAN

This one is done barefooted, standing at arm's length away from the wall. Keeping your back and legs straight, and your heels flat on the floor, lean forward and try to touch your chest to the wall. Feel the stretch as you hold it for 5 seconds. Relax and then repeat, 5 times over. You can do this one leg at a time or with both together, depending on which feels like the best stretch. When you've gotten really good at this one, put a 1- or 2-inch lift under the ball of your foot—a paperback book will do—and keep stretching.

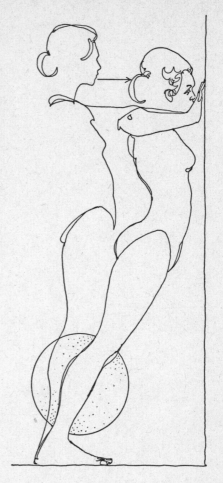

	Groin	Trunk	Shoulder	Elbow
Running	X	X		
Swimming		X	X	
Cycling		X		
Skiing	X	X	X	
Racquet sports		X	X	X
Golf		X	X	X
Bat and ball	X	X	X	
Basketball, volleyball	X	X		
Soccer, football	X	X	X	

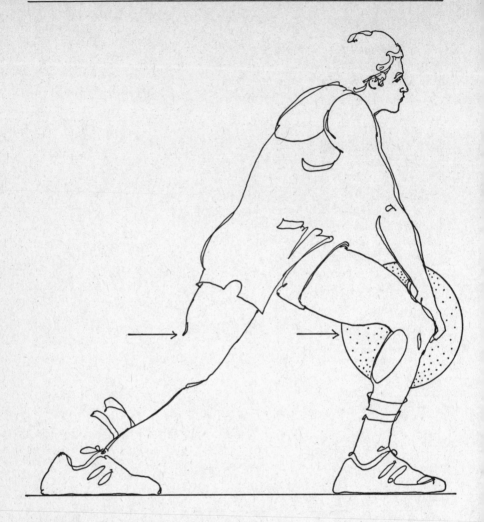

THE RUNNER'S STRETCH

Stand with your right foot 3 feet behind your left. Keep both feet pointed straight ahead. Put your hands on your left knee and lean forward as far as you can, keeping your right heel on the ground. Feel the pull, and hold for 5 seconds. Relax, and then repeat, 5 times for each leg.

SLANT BOARD STRETCH

Build yourself a wooden wedge measuring 3 inches on the high side. Stand on it with your toes pointing up, and feel the pull. This is a passive stretch and should be held for several minutes each day. It seems to be good for the anterior compartment syndrome, and helpful in preventing shin splints.

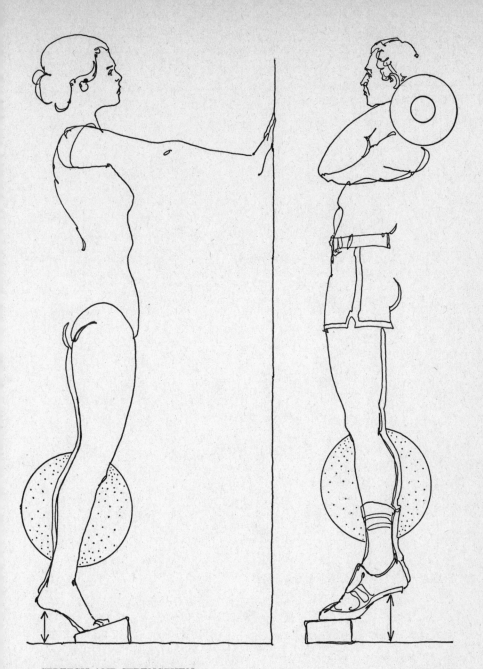

STRETCH AND STRENGTHEN

Stand with the balls of your feet on a piece of 2-by-4 lumber. Hold something that weighs about a quarter of what you do across your shoulders (a barbell, or if you don't have one you can load books into a duffel bag or suitcase). Balancing on the 2-by-4, lower your heels to touch the floor, then rise up on your tiptoes as far as you can. Try to do this 25 times.

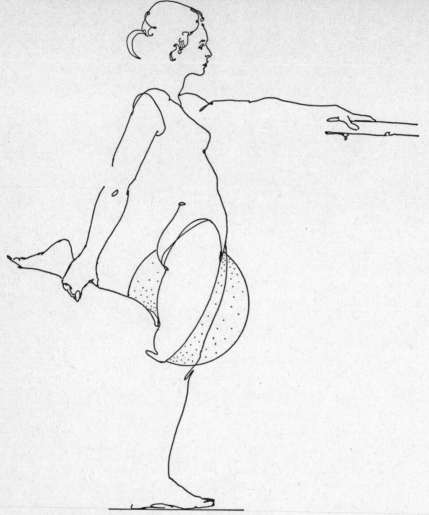

STRETCHING THE QUADRICEPS

The quadriceps are the anterior thigh muscles. They are one of the prime movers in the leg and, along with the hamstrings, work to stabilize your knee. There are many acceptable ways to stretch them.

STANDING STRETCH

Stand on one leg while you hold on to something for balance. (Or balance yourself with one arm outstretched and both eyes focused on a blade of grass or a spot of carpet nearby.) Grab your ankle with one hand and bring your heel to your buttocks. The trick here is to keep your trunk straight and to extend your hip as far as possible. Feel the pull in the front of your thigh, and hold for 5 seconds. Relax and then repeat, 5 times for each leg.

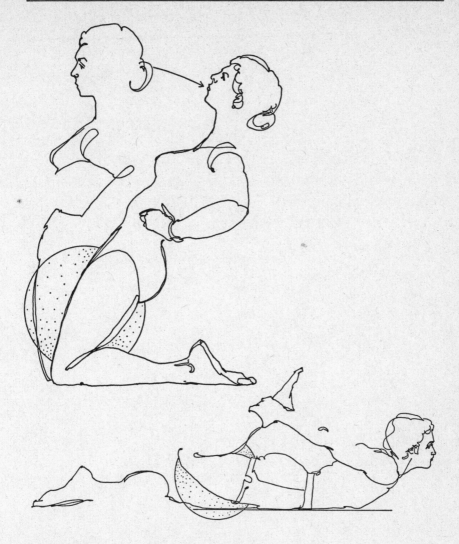

ON YOUR KNEES

Sit on your knees with your feet pointing straight out behind you, toes down. Keeping your trunk straight, slowly lean backward. Find a spot that's comfortable but that stretches you, and hold it for 5 seconds. Relax and then repeat 5 times.

LYING DOWN STRETCH

Lie face down. Keeping your hips on the floor, bend one knee so that you can grab your ankle. Bring your heel up to your buttocks, feel the stretch, and hold for 5 seconds. Relax and then repeat, 5 times for each leg.

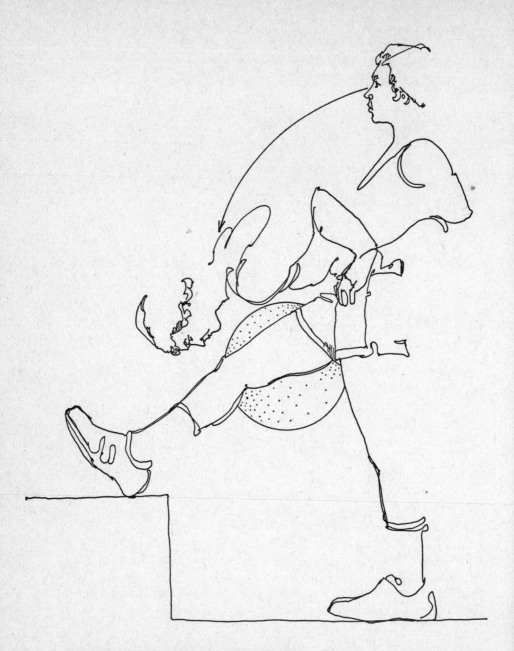

STRETCHING THE HAMSTRINGS

A pulled hamstring is a very common sports injury. Tight hamstrings are easy to identify, though, and shouldn't be difficult to stretch out.

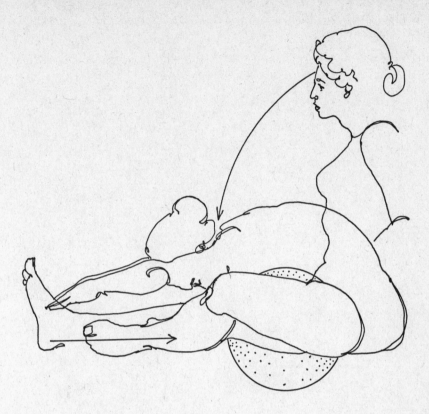

THE HURDLER'S STRETCH

This is an effective exercise but you have to start out slowly, and build it up gradually. Put your leg up onto a steady object, such as a fire hydrant, a bench or a chair. Point your toes straight up, keep your knee straight and lean forward to touch your ankle. Don't bounce down, but stretch gently and breathe your way down. When you can put your nose on your knee, switch the exercise to something higher. Hold this stretch for the usual 5 seconds, and repeat it 5 times.

YOGA STRETCH

Sit with one leg straight out in front of you, toes pointing up. Bring the opposite heel as far as you can toward your crotch, keeping that thigh flat on the floor. Then, with your knee straight, gently lean forward, trying to reach your ankle and put your forehead on your shin. Feel the stretch and relax. Repeat 5 times for each leg.

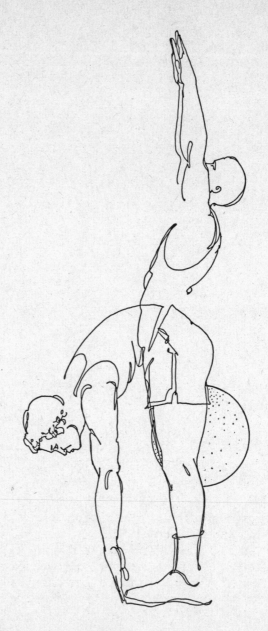

THE TOE TOUCH

   Stand straight, with feet slightly apart. First stretch your arms straight up overhead, reaching for the sky. Then slowly bend forward to touch your toes. Come as far as you can, without bouncing. Relax, feel the stretch, hold for 5 seconds. Repeat 10 times. (Avoid this if you have any back problems.)

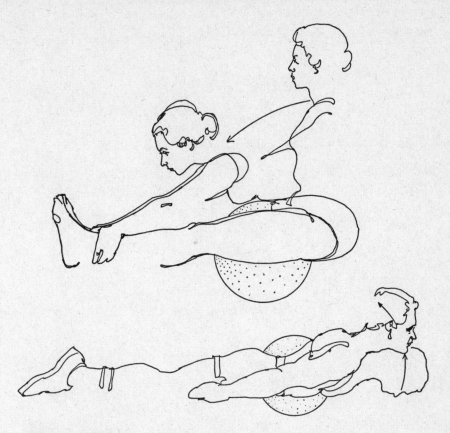

SITTING STRETCH

Sit down with your legs together in front of you, your toes pointed up. Gently stretch forward and try to grasp your ankles. Keep it gentle, don't bounce. This will help stretch your lower back too. Hold 5 seconds. Relax, repeat 5 times.

STRETCHING YOUR TRUNK

Tense, tight trunk muscles contribute to backache and sideaches, and keep you from feeling relaxed and in control.

PRONE STRETCH

Lie face down on the floor with your arms at your side. Raise your head and shoulders off the floor as far as you can. Hold for 5 seconds. Relax and repeat 5 times. Then, keep your legs straight and lift both of them off the floor. Relax, repeat 5 times.

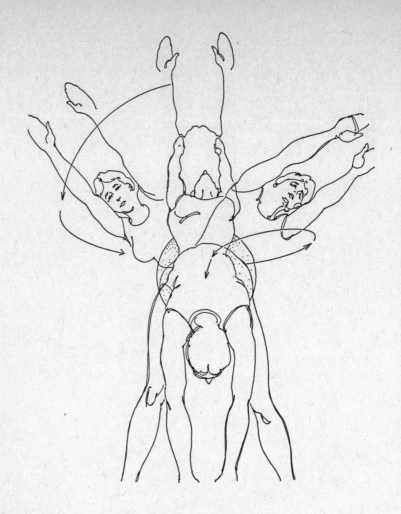

TRUNK STRETCH

Stand with your feet spread to shoulder width. Stretch your arms as high above your head as you can. Keep your torso straight and bend to the right, then backward, then to the left as far as you can, and finish the cycle by reaching forward to touch your toes. Repeat 5 times going to the right, then 5 times to the left.

TRUNK ROTATION

Stand up, legs apart, with your arms outstretched at your side. Twist around each way as far as you can 10 times.

SIDE REACH

Stand with legs apart. Keep your feet flat on the ground, arms relaxed at your side. Keep your torso in line and lean to each side as far as you can, 5 times each way. You should feel the stretch in your lateral hip muscles.

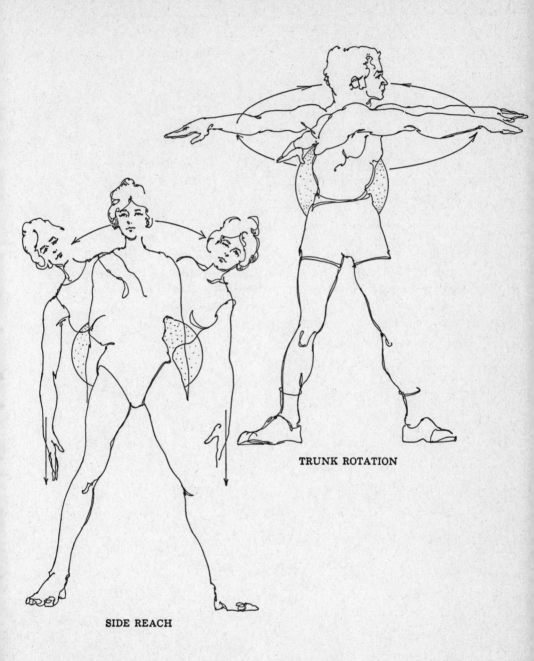

TRUNK ROTATION

SIDE REACH

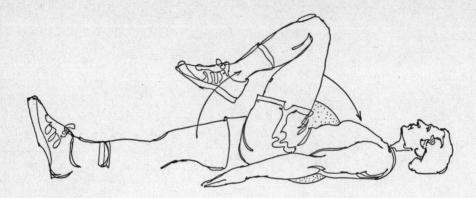

LOW BACK

Lie on your back with knees bent and feet flat on the floor. Pull one knee to your chest and hold it as tight as possible. Keep the opposite leg on the floor. Alternate legs 5 times each, feeling the stretch in your lower back. Then pull both knees to the chest 5 times.

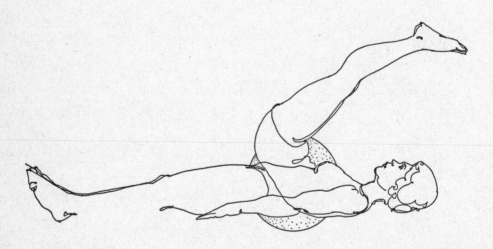

UPPER TRUNK

Lie flat on your back. Bring both legs up and over the head, with the legs as straight as you can get them, and touch your toes to the floor behind your head. Feel the stretch, breathe and relax. Repeat 5 times.

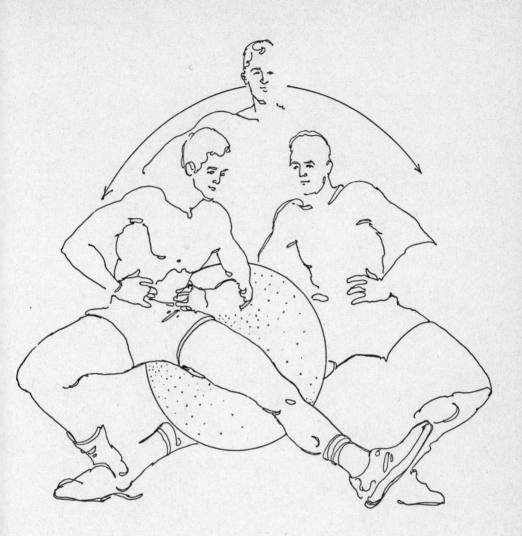

STRETCHING THE GROIN

GROIN STRETCH

Stand with your feet as wide apart as possible. Keep your toes pointed straight ahead. Bend your right knee, roll over onto the inside of your left foot, and lean as far as you can to the right. Feel the stretch in your inner thigh area. Then go to the left as far as you can. Repeat 5 times each way.

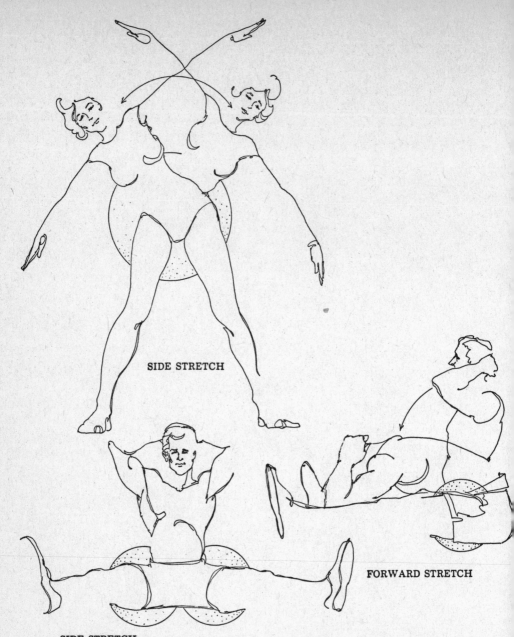

SIDE STRETCH

FORWARD STRETCH

SIDE STRETCH

Stand with legs spread as wide apart as possible. Hold arms out at side, torso straight, and lean over to the right as far as you need to to feel a stretch in your inner thigh. Repeat 5 times on each side.

FORWARD STRETCH

Sit down with your legs spread in front of you as wide as possible. Bend forward, trying to touch your forehead to the floor. Hold the stretch for 5 seconds, relax and then repeat 5 times.

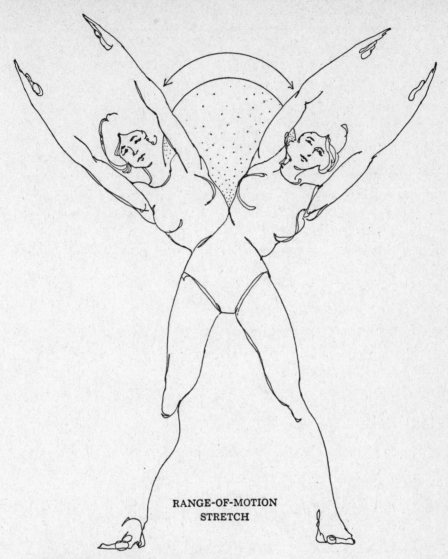

RANGE-OF-MOTION
STRETCH

STRETCHING THE SHOULDER

In normal, everyday activity, you seldom raise your arms above your head, but you frequently do in sports. If your muscles are not stretched out and ready, you can pull or pinch something.

RANGE-OF-MOTION STRETCH

The idea is, very simply, to work your shoulder muscles so your arms swing up and over and around your head and body, through their entire range of motion. Keep breathing, and keep stretching, in all directions for a few minutes.

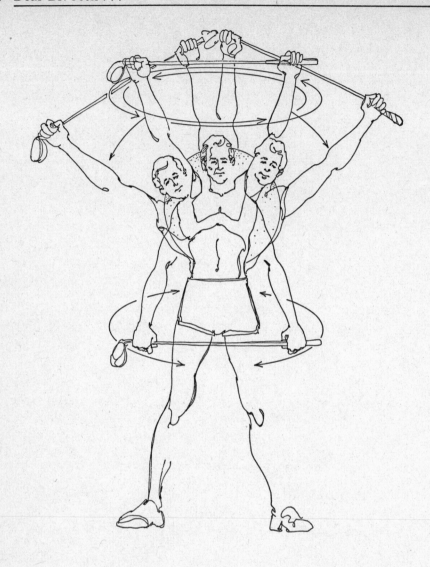

STRETCH WITH CLUB, POLE OR RACQUET

Hold a golf club, a tennis racquet or a ski pole out in front of you lengthwise, one hand at either end of the handle. Bring it as high as you can over your head, and concentrate on stretching upward, toward the sky. Reach backward with it, then move from side to side, and around your back, too. Twist it around so one end is pointing forward, and the other back. Do a series of 5 stretches each way. Then hold the club behind your back and stretch each way as far as you can, 5 times.

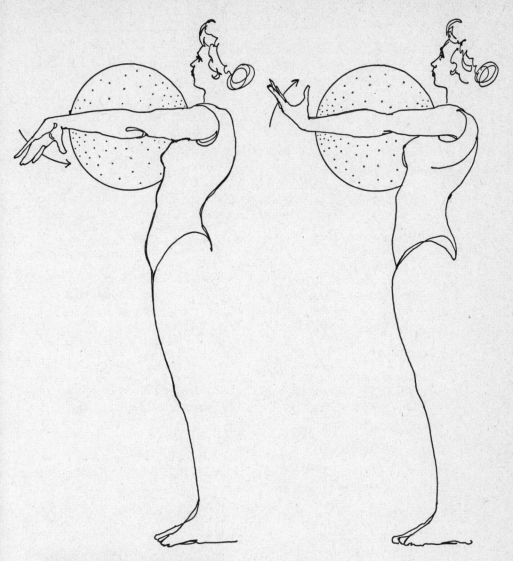

STRETCHING THE ELBOW

These exercises are geared to racquet sport players who need to stretch out the muscles affecting the elbow. They will help prevent tennis elbow.

EXTENSOR STRETCH

Hold your arm out in front of you, palm down, elbow straight, fingers extended. Bend your wrist down as far as you can, and use the other hand to gently stretch it even further. Feel the stretch and hold for 5 seconds. Relax, and repeat 5 times for each arm.

FLEXOR STRETCH

Hold your arm out in front of you, palm up, elbow straight, fingers extended. Bend your wrist down, fingers pointing toward the floor. Use the other hand to gently increase the stretch. Hold for 5 seconds, 5 times for each arm.

HOW FLEXIBLE ARE YOU?

Tight muscles pull and tear; loose, flexible muscles stretch under stress. Athletes need to be very flexible if they want to perform at their best and to avoid the majority of sports injuries. How flexible are you? How much (more) time do you need to spend warming up your muscles before you play? Here's a simple test to help you measure your flexibility.

CALF MUSCLES

Sit on the floor with your legs stretched out in front of you, knees straight and toes pointed straight up. Keep your thighs flat on the floor while you pull your toes up toward your head as far as you can. You should be able to go at least 20° beyond a right angle.

HAMSTRINGS

Lie on the floor with your legs out straight. Keep your right leg flat on the floor, toes pointed straight up. Keeping your left knee straight, raise the leg as high as you can. You should be able to raise it 90°. Repeat with the other leg.

QUADRICEPS

Lie face down on the floor. Bend your knees and bring them to your buttocks. You should be able to touch your heels to your buttocks.

GROIN (ADDUCTORS)

Lie flat on your back, with your legs straight, toes up. Spread your legs as far apart as possible. You should be able to spread them to an angle of 90°.

BACK

Sit on the floor with your knees bent 30°, feet together. You should be able to touch your nose to your knees.

SHOULDER

Lie flat on your back. Move your arm out 90° from your body and bend your elbow so that your forearms are perpendicular to the floor. By rotating your shoulder you should be able to put your palms flat on the floor. By rotating your shoulder the other way, you should be able to put the backs of your hands flat on the floor.

8. Strength

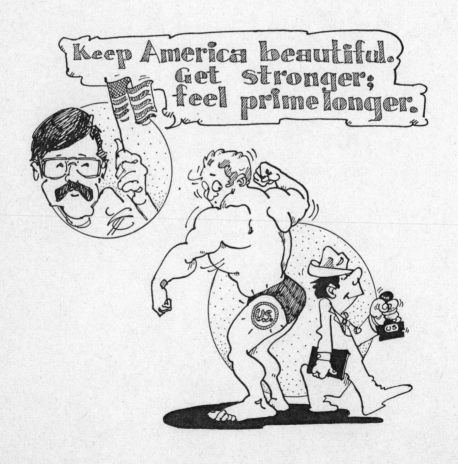

Dear Dr. Jock:

I sprained an ankle very badly last summer playing basketball. I wore a walking cast and took it easy for several weeks. Yet now I find my ankle is still somewhat swollen. And after strenuous exercise even if it's taped my ankle still hurts, mainly on the inside from the top of the ankle all the way down to the instep. Are there any exercises I can do to strengthen my ankle? Thanks for your help.

P.S., Chicago, Illinois

Dear Dr. Jock:

I have been lifting weights lately to help me in basketball. I am 16 and 6'4", 180 pounds. I also have been working on a machine called the "Leaper." It works on isokinetic principles, and is supposed to help your jumping ability. I've stopped using it because I heard that it can hurt your back to the point where an operation is necessary to correct the problem. My friend told me when you push up the machine, the stress exerted on your back was enough to crush the vertebrae together and maybe break them. Is this true? Is the machine safe?

J.C., Lombard, Illinois

Dear Dr. Jock:

I am a 17-year-old girl into bike racing and tennis. I would like to know more exercises for tightening and strengthening my leg and arm muscles. Right now I do sit-ups, jog a mile or two each day, and do push-ups. Anything else I should

J.M.W., Carmichael, California

Might may not make right, but in sports it's essential. Strong muscles protect you against injuries and help you perform more efficiently. No matter what your age, your sex or your stature, sooner or later, if you're serious about fitness, you're going to need to know about strengthening exercises. Muscles that have been taught endurance will keep you going longer and feeling stronger, with less pain. If you're a runner frustrated by endless knee problems, you may be able to find a real measure of relief by working out with a weight boot. The stronger you make your quadriceps and hamstrings, the less stress and strain the knee has to endure. To avoid or at least postpone a crippling case of tendinitis, smart tennis players will exercise to build up important muscles in the forearm and wrist. The better the arm is prepared to absorb the shock and return hard-hit tennis balls, the less pressure is applied specifically to the vulnerable tendon attachment on the elbow of the playing arm.

Besides making good sense in preventing injury, strong muscles allow you to move more quickly, jump higher, start faster and whip forehand kill shots into the front corner. You don't have to be strong to be a sensational golfer, but the stronger you are, the more control you have over your muscles, the more responsive they are to the subtleties.

Any athlete will benefit from ten minutes a day spent developing stronger muscles. Men seem always to have known this almost instinctively. Women athletes, though they have been a little behind, are catching up quickly, and there's every good reason why they should. We frequently hear from women runners and tennis players, and from the mothers of young gymnasts, among others, who are worried that any female working with weights will wind up with unsightly bulges, and big, bulky biceps.

That's not true; muscle bulk is determined by the presence and amount of male hormones and unless you're a woman possessed, willing to subject yourself to the dangers and risks involved in male hormone shots (remember the flap at the last Olympics and those East German women swimmers with shoulder muscles the size of most women's thighs?), you've got nothing to worry about.

Yes, a proper strength program will shape up your body and may put a few new curves on you in places you normally used to just put perfume, but that's certainly nothing to worry about. Indeed, setting those kinds of curves for yourself is something you should be proud of.

The only caution about strengthening your muscles is that the stronger they are, the more you will have to work on flexibility because strong muscles are more easily injured than weak, flexible ones, since they tend to be tighter and more contracted even at rest. That's why weight lifters and other body beautifuls don't do themselves any favors when they concentrate on nothing but strength, and forget about flexibility. Some of them get so muscle-bound that they can't play sports at all without risking a muscle pull.

GETTING STARTED

If you are toying with the idea of strengthening exercises, start out by setting yourself a goal. If you're a tennis player, give yourself a month to put some pizzazz in your serve. If you're a runner, your goal will probably be to get rid of those nagging leg pains by tightening up your quadriceps and hamstrings. Give yourself six weeks of weight work and see what a difference it makes. No matter your sport, you can improve it tremendously if you make up your mind to strengthen the appropriate muscles.

So think of a goal that suits your sport—and suits your level of accomplishment to date—and write it down, preferably in a fresh, clean notebook. The best behavioral scientists tell us that keeping a goal-oriented journal when we are trying to change old habits or adapt new ones is an excellent way of keeping ourselves on track. Once you have set your goal, write down what exercises you need to do to fulfill it. Whether you are trying to improve a general skill or to come back after an injury, you should begin by thinking about the major muscles you use in that sport. Then find the strengthening exercise in this book (supplemented, if you choose, by others you may have picked up elsewhere) for those muscles. The chart on pages 152–153 will help.

Write down the routine you plan to follow. If there are any questions in your mind about what you should or should not be doing, you should see a qualified coach, athletic trainer, physical therapist, fitness counselor or yoga teacher. To have the desired effect, exercises must be done the right way, and if you don't understand what you're doing, you can really do yourself damage. That's why we don't like to go into too much detail in advising people on weight-lifting programs. You should be shown, in person, how to handle heavy weights. As with all things involving your body, you shouldn't push too far, too fast. Your body will stop you before you go too far wrong in the exercises we've given you (that's the nice thing about pain), but you have to use some caution no matter what sort of strengthening routine you follow. At the very least, you should be sure to do warm-ups *before* you do strengtheners.

Make an entry in your journal each time you work out with weights, even if it's no more than the date and a series of dashes. After a particularly good session, one that seems to breeze by in half the usual time, you'll want to write more. If you were bored and want to quit, write that down. If you felt a headache coming on halfway through, but took five deep cleansing breaths and got rid of it, make a note of that. Keep track to stay on track—it's really just common sense.

When the four weeks or the two months are up, and you're finally ready for that week of cross-country skiing in Vermont, or confident that this time you'll break four hours in the marathon, you'll have to make a decision. Either you can throw away your little notebook, content with what you've accomplished, or you can decide that you feel good enough about working toward that first goal to be ready for a second one. In other words, you must decide whether you want to stop . . . or keep going. Keeping going is the best choice, but you are the one who has to choose.

STRENGTH TRAINING: A FOUR-LETTER WORD—W-O-R-K

You can sign up at the poshest gym in town or take out a membership in a legitimate health club with the latest and best equipment—but if you're not ready and willing to do the work, forget it. Every tower of strength is built on buckets of sweat. If you're not psyched up and ready for some kind of pain, some kind of real effort, no book, no program, no coach in the world will pull you through. To paraphrase the venerable Coach Lombardi, there are no losers in the fitness game; there are only players who quit too soon.

As interest in weight training has risen, so has the variety of programs and equipment available. You can be a better shopper by understanding the three basic ways muscles are built up and strengthened. The three chief methods are isometric, isotonic and isokinetic, and the principle behind all of them is the same: in order to build muscles that are *strong* and *powerful* ("able to leap tall buildings in a single bound") with *endurance* ("able to keep leaping from building to building") they must be loaded to capacity. The way you do that is to apply maximum resistance. And the way to do that is by lifting weights.

This is not a new idea. Indeed, stories abound about Milo, the Bruce Jenner of the 6th century B.C. and perhaps the most famous of ancient Olympic champions. He used to run around the stadium at Olympia carrying a 4-year-old bull on his shoulders. Although it has been known for centuries that resisting weights builds strength, we've begun to make a science out of it only in the past thirty years or so.

Nowadays, strengthening is part science, part big business. Since a weak team is not a winning team, more and more researchers are being paid to look for better ways to measure strength and faster ways to build it. That kind of information trickles down from Human Performance Laboratories like the ones in Denver and at Ball State University that work with the world-class athletes, professional teams and the Olympic competitors, to recreational athletes like you.

Thirty years or so ago, athletes who wanted to build up muscle strength had to depend on free weights: the barbells and dumbbells we usually associate with the strong men in the circus. The new machines you hear about—the Universal Gym, the Nautilus equipment, the Bullworker, the Mini-Gym, the Cybex and so on—are mostly variations on the same theme, based on the same training principle. A doctor named T.L. DeLorme discovered that by lifting a very heavy weight (offering high resistance) a relatively small number of times (low repetition) muscle strength and volume can be increased in specific ways. By lifting a lesser weight (offering low resistance) a greater number of times (high repetition) you can develop muscles so as to increase their endurance.

The routine you choose will depend on your needs, your goals and your sport. If you are getting ready for a ski trip to Aspen, your strength training will not be the same as for someone planning to ski cross-country from geyser to geyser at Yellowstone, who will want to concentrate on endurance.

Power—defined as the ability to move your body suddenly—is partially rate-dependent, and exercise rates are getting more and more attention from researchers in sports medicine. Strength and speed are not synonymous. If you train at a slow rate, using heavy barbells, then the laws of physiology seem to dictate that your body is being adapted to heavy, slow work. That's fine if your sport requires you to be powerful at a slow speed, but it won't do a thing for the racquetball or squash player who is looking to speed up his reaction time on the court. You can see what a sticky issue strengthening is, the deeper you delve into it. But try not to get bogged down in details, or in debate about the respective fine points of various pieces of special equipment. Be strong; develop resistance. First master the basics, and those fine points will take care of themselves.

ISOMETRIC EXERCISES

Put your arms in front of you, palm against palm, and press them together as hard as you possibly can. Really grit those teeth and bear down, both palms pushing and resisting at the same time, using as much strength as you can muster, for 5 seconds. That's an example of isometric exercise. If you could look underneath your skin and observe what was happening to your arm muscles as you do this, you'd see that the muscle is contracted, but it would not appear to be any shorter in length. In an isometric exercise, the length of the muscles does not change. Since there is no motion, no mechanical work is performed.

If you did this exercise faithfully every day, 10 or 15 times a day, you would indeed strengthen the biceps, but—and this is the big drawback of isometrics—you would only be making them stronger in one particular position—in this case, the palm against palm. If you bend your arm further placing your palm flat against your cheek, and do another series of isometrics, you'll see that your palm-against-palm exercises aren't helpful at all. That's because isometric exercises do little or nothing to make your muscles strong through an entire range of motion. They also do little for endurance. Since most sports require that a muscle be strong through the entire range of motion, and that you have a large capacity for endurance, isometric exercises are not a highly productive way of building strength for active players. They can, however, be extremely helpful in rehabilitation. If a knee is in trouble and the muscles around it need to be strengthened so as to protect and support it *without* doing any more damage to the sore joint itself, isometrics are the best thing you can do.

ISOTONIC EXERCISES

Isotonic exercise is what we usually mean when we speak of working out on the multistage machines at a health club or gym. This is the most common kind of exercise program prescribed for sports, and weight lifting is the classic example. In isotonic exercise, as the weight is moved, the muscle shortens and lengthens and work is performed. When you lift a weight, fibers shorten as the muscle contracts; this is known as a concentric contraction. When you ease the weight back down, the muscle fibers lengthen; this is called an eccentric contraction. This letting-down process is also called negative work. Some experts believe that you build strength *more* with eccentric than with concentric contractions—which is why you should pay just as much attention to the going-backward portion of a bent-leg sit-up as you do to the coming-forward part.

In pure isotonic exercise, the weight or resistance stays the same throughout the entire range of motion—which leads to some of the drawbacks in isotonic exercising. Say you're trying to lift a 75-pound barbell or do wrist curls with a 5-pounder. Once you have overcome the inertia of the weight with the first muscle contraction, you can continue to move it to where you want it—back and forth—with the expenditure of very little extra work. Some investigators say that in pure isotonic work the muscle is actually working only 30 percent of the time. Another drawback is that you can lift only as much weight as the weakest point in your range of motion allows. If you can lift your arm 180°—from your side up to your head—with a 10-pound weight, but can lift it only as high as your shoulder with a 20-pound weight, that limitation is called your "sticking point." Don't feel bad about it—everybody has one, and if you didn't, you wouldn't need to do strengthening exercises.

For a long time, gyms and health clubs relied strictly on isotonic equipment that offered a constant weight throughout the entire range of motion—dumbbells, barbells and so on. When Universal Gyms first came on the market, they were simply glorified versions of the pure isotonic principle. Since it is now known that the strength of your muscles will vary at different angles of flexion, newer generations of isotonic equipment have come along that vary the resistance throughout the entire range of motion. This innovation is proving very effective in building muscle strength faster and more easily than before.

Major manufacturing companies supplying gyms and health clubs with "dynamic variable resistance" equipment of this kind include Nautilus, Mini-Gym and Universal Gym. Each system has its supporters and its critics and this is not the place to go into the fine points of them all.

If you are thinking about joining a gym or health club, at the very least you should look for one that offers variable resistance equipment. Talk to the person in charge before you sign on, however, and don't sign until you're sure they know what they're talking about. If they can't make you understand clearly how their equipment works, don't be so sure they understand it themselves. And if you don't have the time or the money or the inclination to join a private club, you can work wonders with your muscles right at home, using your own body as weight.

ISOKINETIC EXERCISE

Isokinetic exercise is the third way to build muscle strength, and the least accessible one to the average jock-in-the-street. With isokinetics, you don't lift a weight, you provide resistance to a lever that is moving at a constant speed. Maximum force can be exerted against the lever at all points in the range of motion; this is termed "accommodating resistance." Since you don't have to waste any energy thinking about the speed of the lever (it's preset and can be adjusted to fit the needs of the athlete), you are free to concentrate all your efforts on resisting the lever. As you exercise, you both push and pull against the lever and you get to exercise antagonistic muscle groups (the quadriceps and the hamstrings, for example) at the same time. Strength programs should always exercise opposite muscle groups, since muscle balance is necessary for maximum performance and protection against injury. Since the speed can be adjusted, some people see high-speed isokinetic work as the fastest way to build strength for sports. That's why you'll read about pro stars performing rehabilitation workouts with the Cybex, the Orthotron or the Fitron, an isokinetic stationary bicycle. One of the nicest things about working out on an isokinetic exerciser like a Cybex is that you can actually see the progress you're making by means of an automatic readout, much like the printout on an electrocardiogram. One week, your ailing knee may register only 100 foot-pounds of torque, whereas after a month of diligent work on the Cybex, you may set the curve all the way to 200 foot-pounds of torque.

The drawback about isokinetic equipment is that no eccentric work is done; also, the machines are expensive, and so complicated that you really need someone who knows what he's doing to run them. They're fine for rehabilitation work, and many sport teams use them for testing strength to identify areas of weakness and plan strength programs.

The Mini-Gym equipment you may have heard about is also reported to be isokinetic, in that there are no eccentric contractions and there is a built-in governor that adjusts the speed as the muscles get stronger or more fatigued. These machines are built to mimic specific athletic movements; for instance, the Leaper is designed to improve jumping or starting ability. It's perfectly safe for people with normal spines. They all exercise multiple groups of muscles instead of isolating groups as other devices do. If you want to know more details about them and their use you'll have to look elsewhere.

The important thing to remember about all such equipment is that it works if *you* are willing to work. Don't get suckered into joining some phony health club that offers nothing but some shake-'em-up hip belt massagers or those automatic tushy-roller machines you sit on and jiggle. Not long ago, a nice lady from Orange, California, who signed herself "Thank You Very Much" wrote to us about what she thought was a real brainstorm. Instead of paying so much money to her health club for the privilege of getting her flab jiggled about by a bunch of vibrating machines, wouldn't she do just as well sitting on top of a washing machine while it was set on the spin cycle? (No, we're not making this up.)

"It sounds like a novel idea," she wrote, "and much less expensive than those machines." We had to tell her that her idea just didn't wash. Either routine was essentially worthless, since it didn't require her muscles to do any work. We suggested she forget spin cycling and stick to bicycling.

THE DR. JOCK GIVE-YOURSELF-A-LIFT PROGRAM

Why you want to get stronger is your business, but *how* you do it is ours. We want to make it as safe and simple for you as possible, which is why we recommend strengthening exercises that don't depend on fancy equipment or high-priced club memberships. Fitness should be an easy access activity, available to everyone, and so should strengthening. All the weight you need for our program is with you every day. You don't have to run to the gym, or commit yourself to a year of classes. In our program, you frequently are your own best weight. The cost of the equipment we recommend is minimal—a weight boot shouldn't set you back more than $25—and once you understand the basics of how to use it, the chances of your getting hurt by it are slim.

Once again, though, we must emphasize what we've said so often that by now you must believe it—that you must begin every time with a few minutes of gently stretching out your muscles before subjecting them to the hard work of lifting weights. In other words, before you load them up, wake 'em up a little bit—let them know the work is about to begin.

And since you're not just a body, but a mind too, take these few minutes to get all the energy you can muster concentrated on the issue of the moment: to lift, to keep lifting, to lift enough weight to make your muscles stronger, more powerful, with more endurance, but *not* enough to aggravate the tender tendons that attach to the muscles, not enough to pinch or poke or otherwise mess up the bursas—the delicate sacs that sit over the uneven, protruding ends of a bone so that skin and muscle can slide over them. If you're too exuberant when you lift weights, and if you haven't warmed up properly, these sacs can become inflamed. When that happens you have bursitis, and it hurts. It also could cost you hundreds of dollars in doctors' fees and days off from work and play to get rid of it, so you're better off avoiding the whole thing in the first place. You can read more about how to avoid bursitis in Chapter 4.

How frequently should you work out? We stand by the experts whose research has shown that the most efficient way to strengthen your muscles is to load them up not more than 3 times a week, or every other day. Stretching is something you can and should do every day, but strengthening is different. When a muscle is loaded to capacity and put to work, it breaks down a bit in the process. Then, of course, it is rebuilt—and comes back stronger than ever. But you've got to allow some time in between for that rebuilding process, for the body to attend naturally to its little wounds. If you don't give your body the day of rest it needs to restore itself, in a relatively short time the body will rebel. Your strength will not go on increasing at the same rate, and your risk of being injured will increase.

Before beginning a program of strengthening exercises, you should understand that it will not increase your cardiovascular fitness. It will make you work, and the work will make you sweat, but tests have shown that even in the best strengthening programs—with men and women lifting moderate weights 10 to 15 times in 8 or 12 exercises, with from 15 to 30 seconds of rest between exercises, called circuit training—cardiovascular fitness was not significantly improved. These exercises are geared to making you a stronger, better, safer player. But you must then go out and play to achieve fitness.

We'll outline two kinds of strengthening programs—one that uses weights, and one that primarily uses your body as the weight, working on muscle groups and practical function rather than on single, isolated muscles.

USING A WEIGHT BOOT

One easy way to add weight to leg exercises is with a weight boot. This is simply an iron shoe, weighing 5 pounds, that is strapped to your foot, usually over a pair of sneakers. Extra weights can be added to a

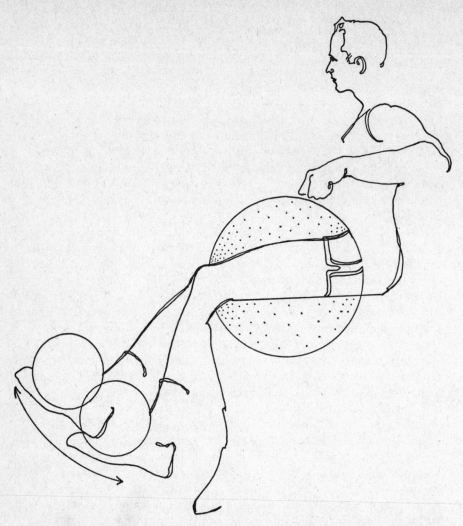

bar that is attached to the heel. You can buy one at a sports store for $25 or so, and under the right conditions it can be useful if you're trying to strengthen or rehabilitate your leg.

There are two problems with using a weight boot: if you don't use it correctly, you can hurt yourself; and it is not sport specific. That means you get strong for lifting the weight boot, but not for skiing or running or tennis. Using it is not a functional exercise, whereas using your body weight to build strength has the added advantage of making you strong in ways that approximate moves you actually make in your sport. (The 90-90 wall lean, for instance, makes you stronger in a position that approximates the bent-knee, half-sitting position you use in downhill skiing.)

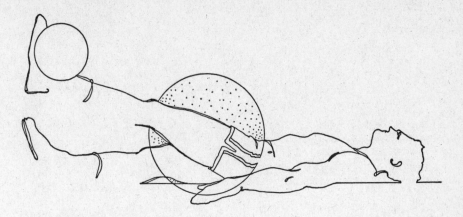

STRENGTHENING THE QUADRICEPS

We can suggest two ways of using the weight boot to strengthen your anterior thigh muscles, the quadriceps. The first is for people who have absolutely no problems with their knees. Strap on the boot, and sit on a high bench or table with your knee bent over the side. Then, sitting upright with your arms at your side, simply extend the weighted knee so that your foot is straight out in front of you. Don't let the weighted leg twist to one side or the other; you could hurt yourself that way. Be sure, too, that you've fully straightened your leg each time you lift, or you won't get maximum benefit from the work. That's because the muscle on the inside of your knee, the vastus medialis, doesn't contract to its maximum unless you get complete extension—and that particular muscle is most important in stabilizing the knee for any kind of sports activity.

If you have knee aches or pains of any sort, your best bet is to use the boot while lying on your back with your knee straight. In this position, you should lift the weighted leg to a 45° angle, then slowly lower the weight to the floor and relax. Be sure to keep your toes pointed straight up and your knee straight. Your kneecap should not move and the knee should not bend, since that action puts undue stress on an already troublesome knee joint.

How much weight should you lift? There are many programs to choose from but one good one combines both strength and endurance. First, you find out—by simple trial-and-error—how much weight you can lift, fairly comfortably, at one time. That's your single lift capacity. Then do a set of 10 lifts with half that amount and a set of 10 lifts with three-quarters that amount. Gradually build up to being able to do a set of 10 lifts with the total amount. The next step is back to square one: find out what your new single lift capacity is, and start all over.

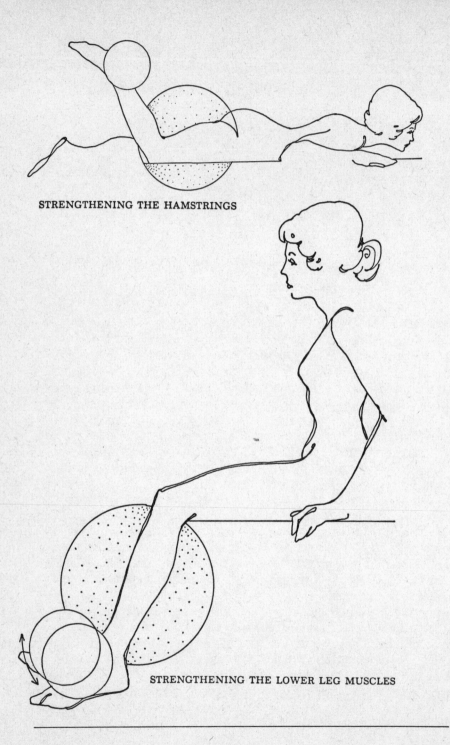

STRENGTHENING THE HAMSTRINGS

STRENGTHENING THE LOWER LEG MUSCLES

STRENGTHENING THE HAMSTRINGS

Lie face down with the boot on your foot. Bend your knee to a right angle and slowly return it to the floor. Find your single lift capacity and do the same sort of program we've outlined for the quadriceps. Kind in mind that your hamstrings are only about 50 to 60 percent as strong as your quadriceps, so you can't expect to use the same amount of weight. It's a good idea to have someone watch from the back as you lift to make sure that you're keeping it straight. If your leg rotates as you lift, you could be hurting yourself. And don't go beyond a 90° angle. With heavy weights, you might lose control and end up getting hurt that way too.

STRENGTHENING THE LOWER LEG MUSCLES

The anterior muscles of the lower leg are important in all sports. They are the ones that pull your toes and foot up, and frequently they're involved in "shin splits." To strengthen them, put on the weight boot and sit on something high so that your leg hangs free. Do 3 sets of 10 repetitions, moving your ankle up and down as far as you can each time. (You really don't need a weight boot for these. A ladies' handbag slung over your foot, or a paint can will work just as well.) Between sets, you should rest for the length of time it takes you to do a set.

DUMBBELLS FOR YOUR ARMS

If you play any of the racquet sports—tennis, squash, racquetball and so on—you will be wise to invest in a pair of hand dumbbells, since strengthening the wrist and forearm is a big part of preventing tennis elbow. We've outlined some specific exercises for this in Chapter 13. Dumbbells can be used by anyone who wants to strengthen the wrist and forearm, no matter what their sport.

You can strengthen your biceps by doing curls. Hold the dumbbells in your hands, palms up. Fully bend your elbows. Then let them down again. Do 3 sets of 10 repetitions. For your triceps, hold the weights in your hands with your elbows fully bent, then straighten your arms, and raise them as high as you can above your head. This will also help strengthen the shoulders.

Other shoulder exercises should be done both standing and lying down. Stand and hold the weights with your arms at your side. Keep your elbows straight and bring your arms backward as far as you can. Then bring them straight forward all the way above your head. Repeat 10 times.

Another shoulder exercise begins from the same position, arms at your side. This time, bring your arms straight out from your side, over

USING DUMBBELLS FOR YOUR ARMS (1-6)

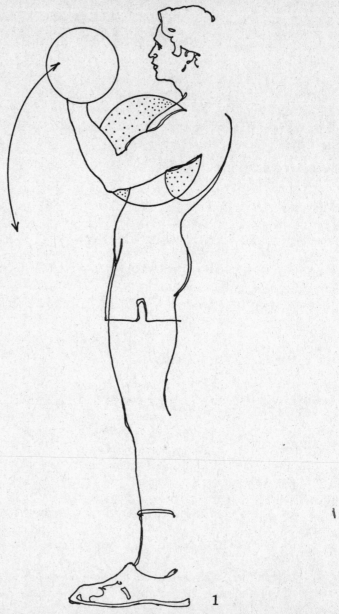

1

your head and then back to the starting position. Repeat this one 10 times, too. Or, you may start in the same position and bring your arms straight out from your side until they are parallel to the floor. Keep them at that height, and move them as far to the front and as far to the

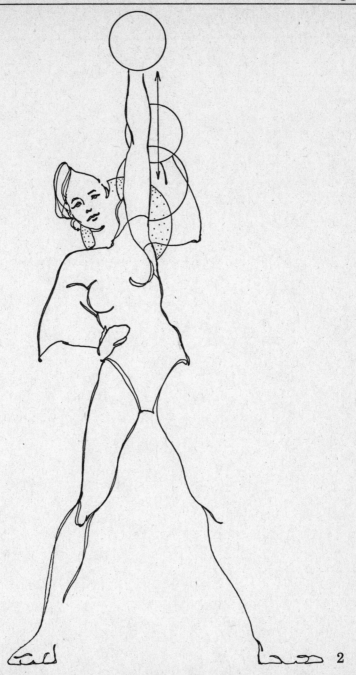

2

back as possible. Repeat the sequence 10 times. Finally, lie down with your arms out at the side, and hold the weights in your hands with the elbows bent. Rotating your shoulders, bring the weights to the floor, all the way down and all the way back. Repeat 10 times.

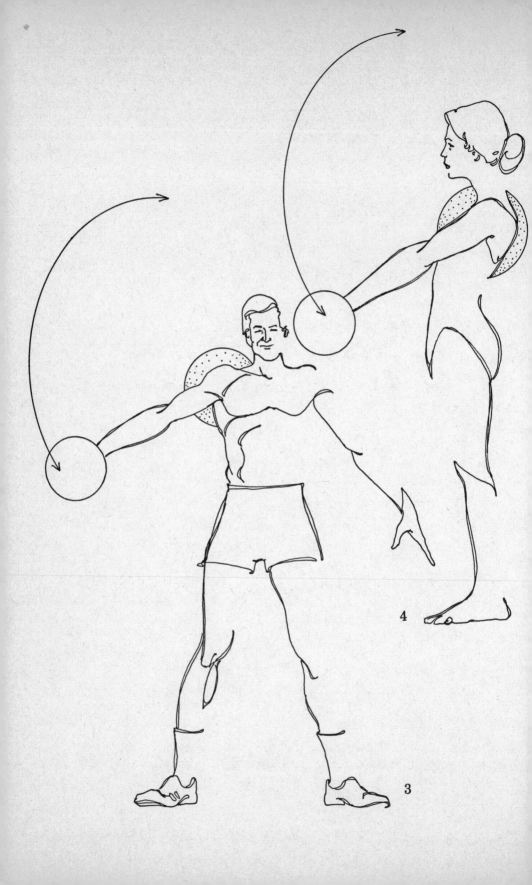

4

3

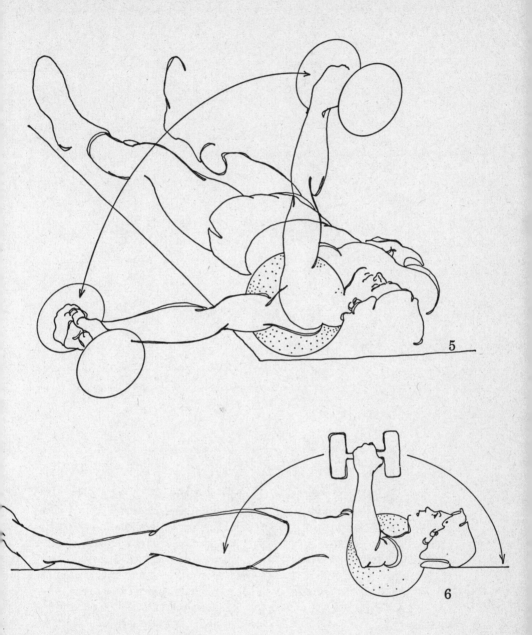

5

6

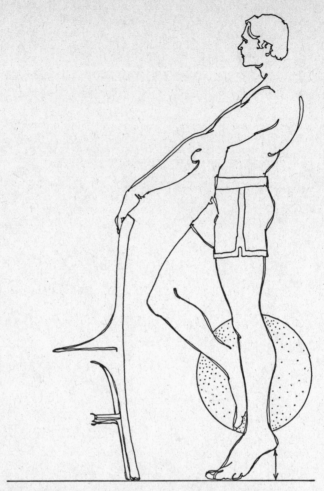

AN EASY, AT-HOME STRENGTH PROGRAM

There are all kinds of strengthening programs. The best, naturally, is the one that has been tailor-made for you, taking into account your own weaknesses and your own needs. A program designed to rehabilitate a weak knee after surgery will be different from one geared to the healthy athlete who wants to improve strength, speed, agility and performance. Sometimes the exercises overlap, sometimes not. The important thing for you to understand is that the series of exercises we recommend are geared to improving your strength in a functional manner. Think about your sport, how your muscles move and function in your sport, and you'll understand why we are focusing on strengthening muscle groups rather than isolated muscles. Strengthening isolated muscles is most helpful in the early stages of a rehabilitation program; otherwise, it's best to talk about functional strength, functional recovery.

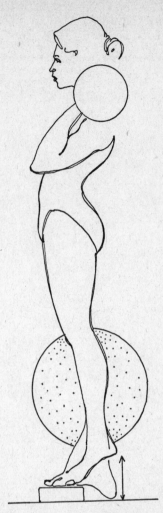

STRENGTHENING YOUR CALVES

Single-leg toe raises. Stand on one leg with the other foot off the floor. You can hold onto a table or the back of a chair for balance. Keep your knee straight and rise onto your tiptoes as high as you can, then return to the ground. Calf muscles of normal strength should permit 10 repetitions. Do as many as you can with each leg.

Toe raises, both legs. This calf-strengthener requires a 2-by-4 and a weight. You can use a barbell equaling 25 percent of your body weight if you have one; otherwise, load up a suitcase, book bag or duffel bag with books, bricks or sand. Stand with the balls of your feet on the 2-by-4. Hold the weight across your shoulder (this is where using a suitcase can get a little tricky). Let yourself down until your heels touch the floor, then rise up onto your tiptoes as high as possible. Do 3 sets of 10 repetitions. This exercise combines stretching and strengthening, and it is particularly good for shin-splint sufferers. Add weight in 5-pound increments every time you master a level.

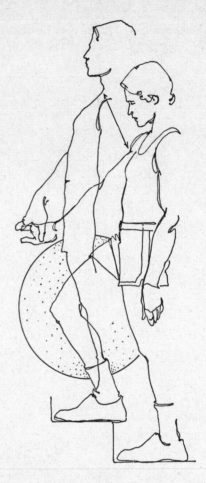

FOR LEG STRENGTH AND AGILITY

Step-ups. Step-ups develop functional strength in all the leg muscles and should help with your jumping ability, too. Start on a stair step where you can hold the railing for balance if necessary. Place one foot on the step. Step onto the step with the other foot, and then back down. Simple enough? Make sure to straighten your knee fully and hold it for a count before you step back down. The vastus medialis, the muscle on the inside of your thigh at the knee, which is a primary stabilizer for the whole knee, gets the full benefit of the workout when you fully straighten your leg at the knee. Aim for 25 repetitions. When you can do them easily, do your step-ups onto a stable bench or chair 18 inches high. These exercises are most valuable for your calf muscles, quadriceps and hip extensors, the leg's primary power muscles for sports.

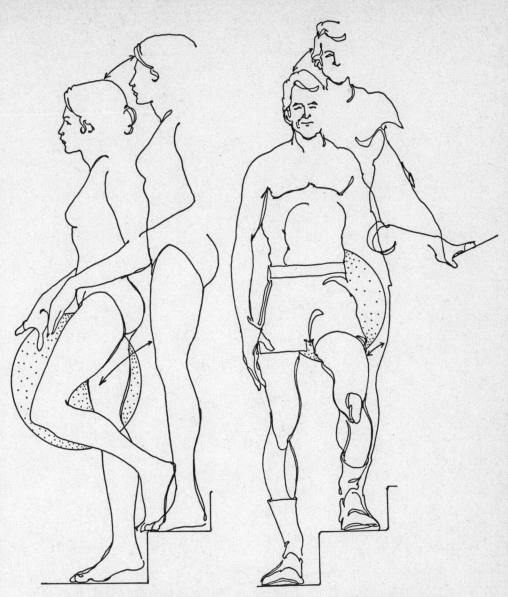

Reverse step-ups. By turning around and doing backward step-ups you can strengthen your hamstrings, too. Reverse step-ups should be done on a stair step since you'll need the railing for balance. Again, aim for 25 repetitions but don't push too hard.

Side step-ups. It's back to the stairs again to strengthen the hip abductor, called the gluteus medius. This is the muscle that allows you to balance on one leg, and it's an important one in all sports. Stand sideways to the stairs. Step up, extend your leg fully, hold it for a count, and step back down. Working one leg at a time, do 25 repetitions if you can.

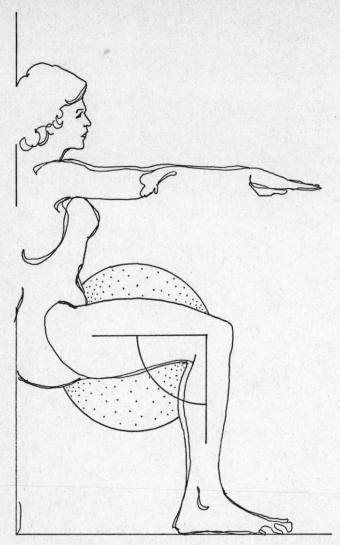

The 90-90 wall sit. This is a very important exercise for skiers. It is an isometric, done in the classic half-sitting ski position and should be a big help to you in maintaining this position and improving your form and control. Stand with your feet 18 inches from the wall. Lean back against the wall and slide down until your hips and knees are bent at right angles. Then rise up onto your tiptoes. Hold that position as long as you can. Time yourself with a watch and try to increase the time by 5 or 10 seconds each day.

Climbing the stairs. This is not a good exercise for anyone who has knee problems, but it's an excellent functional exercise if you don't,

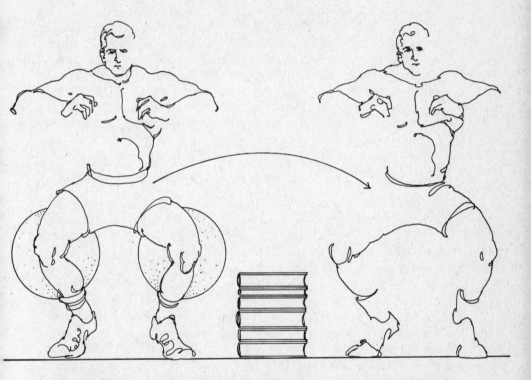

and if you want to avoid knee problems in the future. Begin by walking up several flights, and increase the challenge gradually. You can go from a walk to a run, from one step to two, from five flights to fifteen. This is a simple exercise to fit into your day, and it's also especially good for improving your strength, power, agility and endurance.

The bench jump. This is another good exercise for building power and agility. Stand beside a book and jump over it sideways, back and forth, about 25 times. This should be easy. Now make it tougher for yourself by adding more books to the pile, until you're able to use a box or 18-inch bench. By then you'll be jumping with more confidence.

STRENGTHENING YOUR STOMACH MUSCLES TO PREVENT
BACK PROBLEMS

Bent-knee sit-ups. Everyone should be doing some bent-knee
sit-ups every day. They strengthen the abdominal muscles and give
the best possible protection against back problems. Most of those are
really weak-abdominal-muscle problems. The best way to do sit-ups is
to lie on the floor with your knees bent and your feet flat on the floor.
This flattens your back, relieving the strain on it and at the same time
relaxing your hip muscles, so that your abdominal muscles do more of
the work. Don't do sit-ups with your knees straight and your legs flat
on the ground. Fold your arms across your chest so you're not boosting
yourself up with them. Try to begin from the sitting-up position. Sit
back as far as you can keep control, and return to the sit-up position.
Remember to keep breathing, stay relaxed. You should also alternate
directions as you come up. First, sit straight up and lower yourself
straight down. Then twist gently to the right as you sit up and lie
down; then twist to the left as you sit up and lie down. This will help
strengthen the oblique muscles on the side of your trunk. The stronger
these muscles are, the less strain there is on your back. You should be
able to do 25 sit-ups and 50 is better. Some people like to do 75 or more.

STRENGTHENING YOUR UPPER ARMS AND UPPER TRUNK

Push-ups and pull-ups. Why invest in a lot of heavy equipment
when you can greatly improve upper body strength by using your own
body weight? Most of us have been taught push-ups at some point, but
too many of us cheat when we do them—or we don't do them at all.

Lie down on your stomach, and spread your hands apart at shoulder
width. Keeping your trunk straight, push up until your elbows are
straight; then let yourself down until your chest and abdomen almost
touch the floor. Then repeat. Set your initial goal at 10, but aim toward
doing at least 20. Build your strength gradually, but keep on building.
Some men and most women have trouble with push-ups, not because
they're incapable of doing the exercise but because they come to it
without the necessary arm strength. It takes time to develop that
strength, but you will if you just stick to it. Meanwhile, you can do a
modified push-up. Keep your feet and knees on the floor and push up
from that position, being careful not to raise your butt too high in the
air. Push-ups strengthen your triceps and shoulder muscles. If you are
looking for more of a challenge, do them on your fingertips. This will do
wonders for your forearm muscles, and if you're a racquet sports player
it will help you escape the aches and pains of tennis elbow.

Pull-ups are even tougher than push-ups for most people. Most men
can't do 10 and some can't manage even 5. Women, generally speaking,
can't do any; again, not because they are physically incapable, but

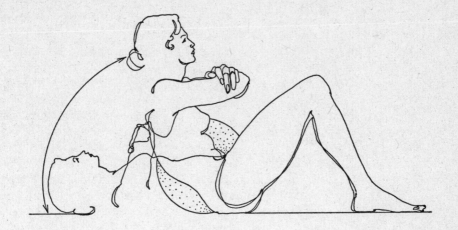

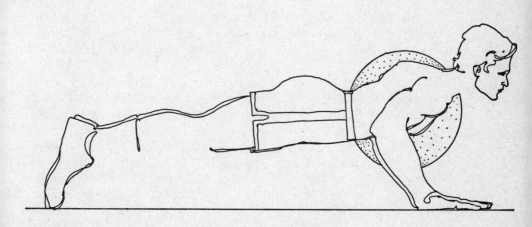

because they've never worked on strengthening their upper arms. To work on yours, buy a chin-up bar and put it in a favored doorway, high enough so that you have to jump to reach it. If it's too low, there's a temptation to cheat by pushing up with your feet. You can get a great stretch by just hanging off the bar, letting your body go limp, working your body loose a section at a time. To do a pull-up, jump up, grab the bar and let yourself down, then pull yourself up until your chin is above the bar. Hold that position while you count, then ease yourself down. Repeat as many times as you can, and don't forget to keep breathing. Alternate your hand positions—palms facing toward you one day, palms facing away from you the next. Doing this will strengthen different sets of forearm muscles. Set your goal at 10, but strive to do more.

Nearly all sports call for changing directions suddenly. To strengthen that skill, run some figure eights. Start with a 20-foot-long figure eight and run it each way 5 times. Then do a 15-foot, then a 10-foot and finally a 5-foot figure eight. Do this 5 times clockwise, then 5 times counterclockwise, doing it as fast as you can.

Tennis players can profit from running down the sidelines, forward and backward, and cutting back and forth front to back, from right to left. Another possibility is the side-to-side shuffle. Run 5 feet to the right, 5 feet to the left. Do it hard, changing directions as fast as you can. Run frontward, backward, sideward—the pattern isn't nearly as important as the practice.

JUMP ROPE FOR AGILITY

Rope-skipping is a fine, all-round conditioning activity for sports, and it's becoming more and more popular all the time. It will make you a more able and agile player, and it will improve your fitness, too, if you stick with it.

Get a rope you can handle easily; the sports store variety with weighted handles are probably the best. Place both feet on the middle of the rope; if the handles reach your armpits you know you have one long enough.

When you jump, choose a soft but stable surface and wear running shoes that are well padded and that support your feet. Socks may help cut down friction and prevent blisters. Don't jump on the bare floor if you can avoid it. Repeated bouncing on the balls of your feet can make them hurt, and whenever that happens to you, you'll have to let your bruises heal. Jumping every other day will give your feet a chance to recover in between.

Jumping rope may be a kid's game but it's hard work for a lot of adults; so start out slowly and build gradually. You may want to start with jumping 15 seconds, resting 15 seconds. Go at a comfortable rate but keep going, increasing your time as you go. When you get to 15 minutes or more, you'll be jumping for joy.

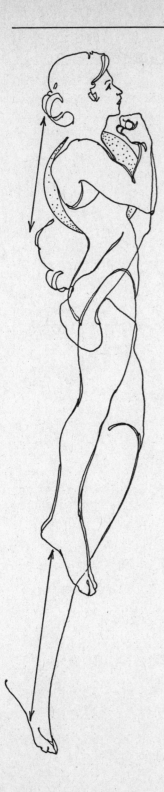

AGILITY DRILLS

We can't stress enough how important it is to strengthen your muscles in ways you are likely to use when you do your sport. The bench jump, for instance, is a big help to skiers, since it works the muscles in the half-crouch position you use when you ski. A baseball player chasing down a pop fly, or a tennis player going into a deeb lob, calls on skill in running backward. The best way to develop it is to practice doing just that.

FIND YOUR SPORT, BOOST YOUR STRENGTH

Strengthening exercises help players perform more efficiently, control their bodies better and keep from being injured. To strengthen your body: (1) isolate the muscle (calf, hamstring, etc.) and use weights; and (2) perform functional exercises. The chart below identifies the muscle groups that most need your attention.

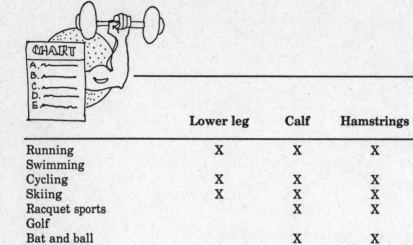

	Lower leg	Calf	Hamstrings
Running	X	X	X
Swimming			
Cycling	X	X	X
Skiing	X	X	X
Racquet sports		X	X
Golf			
Bat and ball		X	X
Basketball, volleyball		X	X
Soccer, football		X	X

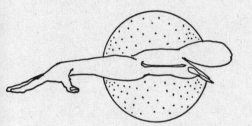 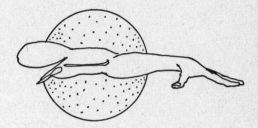

	Quadriceps	Trunk	Shoulder	Elbow
Running	X	X		
Swimming		X	X	
Cycling	X	X		
Skiing	X	X	X	X
Racquet sports	X	X	X	X
Golf		X	X	X
Bat and ball	X	X	X	X
Basketball, volleyball	X	X		
Soccer, football	X	X	X	

III. Enjoy Your Sport, Play It Better

9. Running

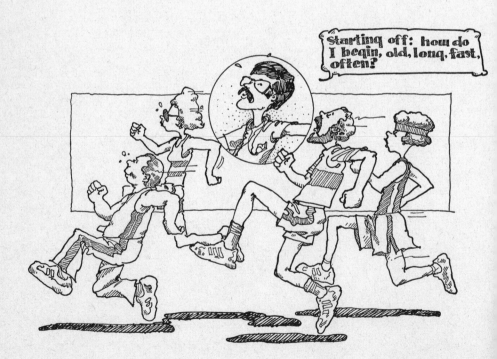

Starting off: how do I begin, old, long, fast, often?

Dear Dr. Jock:

I am a 16-year-old girl and I want to start jogging. I want to get started the RIGHT way, so could you please tell me how long I should jog at first? And how fast, and what should I work up to, and what's the best time of day to jog (considering the Texas heat!) and if there are any special exercises that I should do beforehand to "stretch out"? I've also heard that special shoes are needed for jogging. Can you recommend a good kind? (Like Adidas, London Fog, etc.)

C.C., San Antonio, Texas

Dear Dr. Jock:

I'm a woman, 116 pounds, 27, 5'7", and I've been running for the last six months. I'm slow as molasses sometimes, but I run about 3 miles in 35 minutes. I love running and I'd never give it up for anything in the world, except one thing. I'm pregnant. My gynecologist didn't know if I should continue and said he'd look into it but it's been two weeks and he hasn't called and I don't know what to do. I don't want to stop but I don't want to lose the baby either. My husband suggested I write to you cause he's worried too. What do you say?

M.K., Ft. Wayne, Indiana

Dear Dr. Jock:

I have been running for about one month and have worked my distance up to about 4 miles a day. My problem is after each time I run I have very severe pain around my ankles. The other muscles in my legs are tired, but they don't hurt nearly as much as my ankles. I do a little stretching before I run, wear expensive running shoes, and I walk several blocks home after I run. So what is causing this problem and what can I do about it?

J.C., Highland Park, Illinois
P.S. Please don't tell me to just stop. My own doctor already did that!

Dear Dr. Jock:
I have been running for about three months and I'm beginning to feel a very sharp pain in my knee . . .
N.L., Austin, Texas

Dear Dr. Jock:
Help! Running 5 miles a day makes me feel marvelous except lately I've had to stop because of a severe pain in the bottom of my left heel . . .
O.P., Herkimer, New York

Dear Dr. Jock:
What can I do about "stitches"? I'm a runner who . . .
S.M., Los Angeles, California

Ever since Dr. Jock began, the bulk of the mail has come from runners. And their questions are your questions about how to get started, and how far to go, about the inevitable aches and pains, the fears and myths, the highs and lows that all runners come to know.

Runners, runners and more runners: we've heard from fast runners who want to get faster, from slow runners who want to get fitter, from marathon runners who just want to get to the end. Some of them seem perfectly content with their 3 miles a day; others are running 80 miles a week and don't even think it's enough. We hear from runners of all persuasions and delusions, recreational runners, competitive runners, lone runners, groups of runners, men runners and women runners (pregnant and non).

We hear from California's barefoot runners who do it at dawn on the beach, and Highland Park, Illinois, runners who do it to disco music on a tiny track in the high school. We hear from under-16 runners and over-60 runners, and there was one particular runner from the outskirts of Chicago who always had to urinate in the middle of his run. On the days he ran through the neighborhood streets that sometimes proved awkward. "Is there something I can take?" he wanted to know. A bottle, we suggested.

Runners, joggers, sloggers and schleppers—we hear from them all. Sometimes the questions seem secondary, sometimes they just want to tell us how wonderful they feel since they got hooked on a running program, how the 2 or 5 or 10 miles a day has helped them lose weight, handle stress, stop smoking, meet friends and make sparkling conversation at the dinner table about such wondrous discoveries as the Igloi system and fartlek.

Some who write are just like some of you, hoping to get hooked on running. You've read about the craze, browsed through the best-selling books, poked through all the new running magazines, and you're convinced that running is the answer. You may not even be sure of the question, but there are some 25 million people in the country who will tell you that running seems to be part of the answer. Some of you have even gone so far as to buy a stopwatch and a $35 pair of running shoes, and you write to a doctor, go to a workshop, or read George Sheehan or Jim Fixx or Dyveke Spino or Mike Spino and you want to know the secret. Eventually you discover there is no secret. If not a secret, then what about a few tips: How do I start? What can I do about these awful leg cramps? Why do I get stitches and what can I do about them? Am I better off running shorter and faster, or slower and farther? What about dogs?

Running may, in fact, turn out to be one of the best things to happen to the country in a long time in terms of making millions of people aware of fitness. Runners who stick with it frequently experience something new to them—a feeling of power and energy and self-satisfaction that seems to sustain them and keep them buoyant and joyful when everyone else seems depressed.

When they're not being too obnoxious, runners are admired, and running must share the credit because it is one of the best conditioning sports we know. But runners have their problems too. They're not necessarily serious problems—and the great thing is that you can learn to eliminate about 60 percent of them right off the bat by learning a simple 10-minute warm-up—but the fact is there are problems. And injuries, more injuries to runners than any of us really know. That's because running does put stress on your body, and unless you've spent a little time getting that body prepared for the run, you're risking at least some pain, and possibly an expensive, debilitating sports injury. This chapter isn't intended to scare you, but hopefully it will make you realize that there is a right way to approach running and a way that is . . . well, less right. Certainly, less safe.

Doctors are getting to the point they almost hate to see another malaligned, misinformed runner come into the office. Runners with problems are hard to handle and tough to satisfy because they are looking for an instant cure. They've got two shopping bags filled with running shoes and shoe inserts and no knowledge whatever about what caused their injury. They are hurting and they think it's the doc's responsibility to fix them up. But a doctor—even an experienced specialist with a working knowledge of sports medicine—can only do so much.

Runners' problems could be due to all sorts of things: too much weight, too little motivation or congenital body defects like flat feet or knock knees. It could be bad training habits or a destructive running surface or maybe the runner's foot pronates too much. Most of the time though, the runner has caused his or her own injury.

If you run in ordinary tennis shoes, you're risking an injury. If you run too fast, too hard, before you're in condition, you risk an injury. If you don't stretch out your calf, one day it may rip and tear; if you don't keep your quadriceps and hamstrings flexible and strong, your knee can give out on you—possibly forever. If you don't understand the basics of running and how to keep mind and body supple and relaxed, you're not going to enjoy it as much as you could, and if you're not enjoying your running, the chances are that you're going to quit.

And runners don't want to quit, they want to keep going. But runners are in a peculiar and precarious situation these days. Athletes who don't, won't or can't run anymore are having withdrawal problems.

Not everyone can run, you know, and those people with bad backs or arthritis shouldn't go around feeling underprivileged, deprived or morose. Some bodies just can't take the wear and tear of running—the 1,600 jolts to your body every mile you run. You can cushion the blows, try and fantasize the pain away and master several different bandaging techniques, and you can even work extra hard on your warm-ups, but you still may not be able to make a go of it. And that should be okay, too.

Contrary to popular rumor, there is life after running. There is fitness and calm and mental well-being too, available from cycling, from swimming, from combining racquetball twice a week with several long, fast walks to the office. The world does not begin and end with running; there is Walking, too. Doctors found that fast walkers who walked 40 minutes, 4 times a week, did just as much to improve their cardiovascular system as moderate joggers who ran 3 times a week for 30 minutes a session. So if you're a runner who has to quit because you just can't take the stress and strain, try and slow down to a fast walk and see what happens.

HOW TO BEGIN

You start off the same way you begin any fitness program—with an honest evaluation of who you are and what you want. And if the program is going to work, you'll begin by committing yourself to eight weeks of working at it. Running can seem like very hard work, especially at the beginning. If you're not in condition, and running just seems too hard, you may be better off beginning with some other sport that will build your endurance (such as skipping rope, bicycling or swimming). Or you can start out with a walking program. Whatever way you start, the main thing is that you've got to be good and motivated. If you're not already determined to stay at it for at least two months, with no excuses, you're halfway defeated before you even begin.

The answer is no. You can start running at any age. But there are some cautions:

If you have chronic back pain, running may add to your woes. You should look around instead for the nearest swimming pool. It's possible that later your back will be strong enough to handle the stress.

For people with degenerative cartilage and joint diseases in hip, knee or ankle, running is obviously out of the picture.

If you're 40 or over and wondering whether you might drop dead if you run, by all means have a stress test before you start. If you start out with unresolved fears or anxieties, you'll probably run stiff, and running stiff can increase the risk of getting hurt.

Be realistic. Remember what happened to Lucy, who gave up after that first painful week. You should move at your own pace, find your own rhythm. That's why we don't think beginning runners should start out with a group, nice as it is to have company.

RUNNING FOR CARDIOVASCULAR FITNESS

If your aim is to get into condition, you should follow the guidelines in Chapter 3. That means at least 3, 30-minute workouts a week.

As we've said, anything less than that won't have the effect you need, and more than that may be too much of a risk. There are studies showing that beginning runners who do it 5 days a week experience three times as many injuries as 3-days-a-week runners.

The big problem with running every day is that it doesn't give your body a chance to rest in between. It needs to rest not because you're tired—no, runners report they feel more energetic than ever before—but because it needs that in-between time to heal any minor insults and injuries you might have caused, quite unconsciously, while you were pounding down the track. If you continually abuse your body—neglecting your warm-ups and overusing vulnerable muscles and joints—you are going to cause a breakdown. That's what tendinitis is. You can prevent a lot of running-related sports injuries by not trying to run too far, or too fast. If you prefer to run every day, at least alternate easy days with hard days. And if there are some days your body simply refuses to budge, don't ignore it and force the issue. There is such a thing as body wisdom, and if yours refuses to respond one day, pay attention.

RUNNING HARD ENOUGH TO PRODUCE A TRAINING EFFECT

To have a training effect, you have to run hard enough to push your pulse to between 60 and 85 percent of your maximal heart rate. You can figure out your maximal heart rate by subtracting your age from 220, and then figuring out your goal pulse. If you're 40, for instance, you should try and push your pulse up to approximately 75 percent of 180, to about 135 beats a minute or 23 beats for 10 seconds. Then keep it there for about 15 minutes. (You'll find the chart on p. 33 in Chapter 3 helpful in deciding what your pulse rate should be in order to achieve a training effect.)

It's easy for runners to check their pulse rate during a run. About 10 minutes into the run, put your finger on your throbbing carotid, at the neck under the chin, and watch the sweep hand of your watch for 10 seconds. Multiply in your mind by 6 and you know if you're running with enough intensity.

Most beginners run too hard. Their breathing gets out of control, the heart starts pounding and the lungs feel as though they're being squeezed to death. If this happens to you, slow down. Forget about your pulse and explore the pleasure of running. Don't push yourself so hard, or run so fast, that you're setting yourself up for failure. If you're one of those people who can't run fast, don't let that worry you. Slow running for long distances will get you where you want to go. The main thing is to keep going . . .

RUNNING AT LEAST 30 MINUTES

To achieve that training effect we all lust after, you should keep moving a minimum of 30 minutes a session. At the start, you may want to run part of the way, walk most of the way and pray for a passing pulmotor in between, but don't exercise for any less than 30 minutes. As you get stronger, and in better condition, your body will want to go longer, and that's fine as long as no other complications set in. If you run much less than 30 minutes you're not giving yourself a fair shot at all the benefits of running.

Most everyone has a tough time the first 10 minutes or so. It takes time to get the juices flowing, to shake loose all the pressures of the day and shift over to the sensibility you need to enjoy your running. In the first 10 minutes, you'll probably think of at least three good reasons to stop. "Isn't today too cold to run"? "Is this a bad stitch or is my appendix really about to burst?" "I *can't* run today—I may miss an important phone call . . ." Once you run through those mental obstacles, you can begin to relax. You can notice that the sky has never seemed bluer and that the leaves seem to be turning early this fall and then you can really begin to enjoy your run. If you enjoy your run—and you understand how to keep enjoying it—your chances of getting permanently and safely hooked are wonderful.

What about that high? Runners who have experienced it say it usually doesn't set in until 40 minutes or more after starting out, and sometimes it doesn't happen at all. If you're looking for that kind of euphoric, mystical experience—and more and more runners are, nowadays—the longer you run, the more likely it becomes. But there is a limit to how long and how far you ought to go. We can't tell you what that limit is for you; it's different for every person. If you run too far, you can hurt yourself. Doctors see this happen all the time—an error that comes from exercising no judgment. We can give you guidelines, but it's *your* program. You're the one in charge.

PREVENTING INJURIES

What about the aches and pains and all the medical problems connected with running? Can they be prevented? For the vast majority of these, the answer is yes. It's an easy question to answer; the hard part is getting it to sink in. It's estimated that 80 percent of running injuries are due to inflexibility or overuse—both of which you can do something about.

WARM UP BEFOREHAND

Running strengthens the leg muscles, but it also tightens them. As a result, runners tend to be tighter-muscled than most people. Muscles that don't stretch put extra stress on the tendons. And that can lead to painful, sometimes crippling cases of tendinitis. Also, the older you are, as we've already mentioned, the tighter your muscles become— unless you do something to loosen them up. The first thing a would-be runner can do to prevent injuries, then, is to make a firm commitment to warming up for 10 minutes before starting to run. Ten minutes to stretch the quadriceps, the hamstrings, the calves, the adductors, and to work out any kinks you feel in your trunk, your shoulders, your arms or neck. You'll find the details about all this in Chapter 7.

While you're warming up, really concentrate on your body. Don't just blithely run through some mechanical calisthenics, without focusing on what's happening. Are your calves especially tight today? Do you feel your hamstrings quivering as you stretch them? Don't bounce through your warm-up routine. Go at it smoothly and gently; establish some kind of rapport with the part you're working on. You'll run better as a result.

DON'T STOP COLD

When your run for the day is over, keep your body moving, your blood pumping for another 5 or 10 minutes. Runners who get leg cramps at night or wake up the next day with sore, aching limbs frequently have neglected this important cool-down period.

STEER CLEAR OF OVERUSE

When you're starting out in any fitness program, you must be patient, or you risk getting hurt. We believe in allowing your reach to exceed your grasp, and testing your limits and all that. But if you try for too much, too soon, faster than your body tells you, then you do risk getting hurt. Learn to listen to your body, and it will tell you when it's had enough. Begin by listening to your breathing. Focus on it. In slow, long-distance running, it should be steady, and come easily enough so that you're able to carry on a normal conversation with another runner. To start out, you can do this if you run a little, walk a little, then run a little. This way, eventually, you will build up your endurance. And by conditioning your body, you bring down the risk of getting hurt.

WHAT ABOUT RUNNING SHOES?

One great plus in running is that it's a relatively low-cost sport. You don't have to shell out for costly court time, or buy lift tickets, join a club or invest in expensive equipment. The only thing you shouldn't try to save money on is shoes. Cheap shoes, those that are poorly engineered, with no support or flexibility, can lead to all sorts of foot, ankle, knee and leg problems.

WHAT TO LOOK FOR IN TRYING ON SHOES

The sole should be thick enough to cushion your feet from repeated pounding. Some people prefer the waffle or ripple sole for road running. Your choice will depend on the terrain where you run. You should tell the salesperson what sort of terrain that is. The heel of the shoe should be elevated about one-half inch to relieve the pull on the Achilles tendon. People silly enough to run in high-top basketball shoes can irritate that tendon and cause themselves some painful problems. The heel should be rounded or soft enough to give, rolling your foot forward as the heel strikes the ground. The shoe should be widened at the heel to stabilize the foot when it lands, reducing the chances of turning your ankle. Indeed, the whole shoe should give you that kind of support. A flexible shoe also helps reduce some of the stress on your knee. And make sure there's enough room in the toe so that your foot doesn't jam with every step (a good way of bruising the toes, or even losing a few toenails).

The most important thing, though, is making sure the shoe fits. Don't mistake the #1 ranked shoe or most heavily advertised shoe for what feels right. You've got to find one that fits you and feels comfortable on your foot when you run. This may take some trial and error. To boost your chances of finding the best shoe for you in the least amount of time, be sure to shop in a store that offers a wide range of choices and brands. If shoe width is a problem for you, find out which brands carry extra-narrow or extra-wide shoes. (There aren't many, but there are hopes that the situation may change to meet runners' demands.) Some runners with a persistent fit problem end up having their shoes made for them.

When you go to a fitting, wear the combination of socks you'll be wearing when you run. Some runners prefer no socks at all; but for most people, a thick and thin pair are comfortable, helping cut down on the friction that can cause painful blisters.

WHAT ABOUT ORTHOTICS?

An orthotic is a man-made arch support that slips into your running shoe. You can buy a pair over the counter, or you can go to a podiatrist or an orthopedist and have a pair custom-made. That can be costly—$150 or more. But orthotics can in fact be very helpful to athletes whose feet or legs are giving them pain. The foot is a complex and delicate structure; and if your arch is too flat, some bones are just slightly misaligned, or if you're landing on the outer edge of your shoe and rolling inward, a specialist may be able to advise you about orthotics—preferably a specialist with an interest and experience in sports medicine. But don't think orthotics are a panacea. They can be useful, or they can end up doing the runner more harm than good. If you're in the market for a pair, shop carefully. Don't be afraid to ask lots of questions. And don't expect miracles.

RUNNING PAINS

Runners experience all kinds of pain. It can come from an inflamed Achilles tendon, from a scarred kneecap or simply from tension and boredom. Physical and mental pain are virtually inseparable in many runners' bodies. Pain is an important body signal; and those long-distance runners and other self-sacrificing athletes who keep going by entirely dissociating themselves from their bodies can outsmart themselves into serious injury. On the other hand, many aches and pains are not serious and may best be ignored. What you need to do is to train your body to distinguish between the two, and deal with the situation accordingly. In Chapter 16 we tackle serious sports injuries one by one; that chapter is required reading for every runner who wants to avoid getting hurt. Here, we'll simply mention the kinds of pain a runner may experience.

THE STITCH

This is a notorious pain that many runners know all too well—a cramping, stinging sensation, usually on the right side, above the stomach. There are several theories about what causes a stitch (also called a sidesticker)—gas in the colon, spasms in the diaphragm or running on a too-full stomach, for example. Jack Sinclair, a physiology professor in New Zealand, thinks the cause is a stress or stretching of the ligaments that support the stomach, liver and spleen. The recommended cure, in that case, would be to get pressure off those ligaments. Inhaling and exhaling deeply will help; some runners like pressure-breathing, through pursed lips. You can try bending forward at the waist, putting your hand on the painful spot.' If the pain is really bad, it may help to lie flat on your back, lift your legs over your head and keep them moving as you support your hips with your hands. If you're adept at standing on your hands—or desperate enough to try it—you might succeed in reversing the painful pull that way. You're less likely to develop a stitch if you avoid running until several hours after eating (or vice versa). But if you've been careful and you get a stitch anyway, you may get relief by imagining that cool water is running over the spot that hurts, or by visualizing a thousand tiny hands, all working to massage the pain away. As your overall fitness improves, stitches should become less of a problem.

PAIN AROUND THE KNEE

This is probably the number-one complaint of runners, and the causes of it are legion. It could be a patellar tendinitis—the result of overuse, leading to inflammation of the tendon that attaches to the inferior tip of the kneecap. If you're a woman with a tendency to be knock-kneed, you could be running with your kneecap off track. See Chapter 16 for more about these problems.

SHIN SPLINT

This isn't a specific ailment, but the term runners use for any pain in the front of the leg, between the knee and ankle. Pain of this kind may be the result of overuse. It could come from fallen arches, flat feet, an uneven gait or improper shoes. It may be that one leg is longer than the other, or there may be a stress fracture, the kind that doesn't show up initially on an X-ray. Often, it's the result of not warming up properly. All of this, once again, is discussed at length in Chapter 16.

Sometimes pain in running comes from muscles that are simply too tense. Until you know what you're doing, it may happen that the harder you try to relax, the tenser you get. If you're running and feeling very tight, take a few minutes to shake yourself out. Let your shoulders go limp, let your arms flap and imagine that your legs are turning into smooth, rich, free-flowing honey. That's what is called visualization; it can help you to cope with pain if you're willing to take the little leap of faith that's required. Some runners find they can cope with pain of this kind—and other kinds too—by deep abdominal breathing exercises, similar to the ones that are taught in natural childbirth classes. Biofeedback research has shown that it's possible to train yourself to isolate and relax one muscle at a time. You'll find the details about all these methods in Chapter 5, on body-mind conditioning.

PAIN AFTER YOU RUN

Swelling is a prime cause of this. Minor aches and pains can be treated by applying ice to the sore spot for a period of 15 or 20 minutes—3 or 4 times a day if necessary. Don't use heat on sore muscles; it only increases swelling. Aspirin is helpful in cutting down inflammation, as well as being a remedy for pain—but it's a remedy you shouldn't abuse by turning it into a habit. Naturally, if the pain persists or is disabling, you should see a doctor.

WILL I GIVE MYSELF ARTHRITIS?

Runners sometimes wonder aloud whether they are wearing out their joints by running 60, 70 or 80 miles a week, or even more, month after month. We don't actually know what the long-term risks are, though we believe that the long-term benefits of a running program, within limits, outweigh those risks. More research is needed before the question can be finally answered.

In the meantime, if you start feeling some inexplicable pain, don't assume that your running days are over. Use your common sense. Listen to your body and look for what might be wrong. Are you wearing the right shoes? Have you worn them so long that they've started falling apart? Do you have a tendency toward flat feet? Are you conscious of landing solidly on your heel, and gently rolling forward onto your toes when you run? Are you really taking enough time to stretch and warm up the quadriceps, calves and hamstrings before you run? Try to understand what's happened. Use this book to educate yourself.

TO RUN OR NOT TO RUN?

Every runner who's hurt has the same question: do I have to stop running? The answer depends on your injury, your drive, your tolerance for pain. If your sore knee or aching foot is a result of overuse or inflexibility—as most injuries are—then you can continue running as long as you like. You can self-treat with ice and aspirin and if the pain doesn't get so intolerable it ruins all your fun, you can run and not worry that you are making the condition worse. You're not. In fact, by the time you're feeling pain, the body is already busy healing itself, but that takes time. It could take weeks or months, depending.

Some injuries should not be run on. If it's something mechanical, like a torn Achilles tendon or a ripped calf muscle, you can't continue.

If it's an eroding case of chondromalacia, you'll have to stop because running will make it worse. That's why you frequently need a doctor, to make a proper diagnosis.

WHAT ABOUT CORTISONE?

Judiciously administered, a single shot of cortisone may ease the pain. But be wary. Cortisone may also involve harmful side effects, and is best avoided altogether. If that one shot doesn't work, change your program. Don't get more injections.

FOOD AND DRINK FOR RUNNERS

The rules about eating we should all follow apply to runners: lots of carbohydrates, easy on the fats and red-meat protein, stay away from sugar and processed foods, eat lots of bran, natural grains and fresh produce. If, by some twist of fate or force of habit, you're getting a balanced diet that provides all the vitamins, minerals and other nutrients your body needs, you don't need supplements. If you take time out to get the advice of a nutritionist, you may be surprised to learn how many deficiencies there are. Don't rely on your regular medical doctor to advise you—the chances are that his medical training neglected nutrition. Chapter 6 will help you develop your own nutritional awareness.

What about the so-called energy boosters—Tiger's Milk, ginseng, vitamin E or C or B6? What about those special high-energy capsules? Psychologically, you might get a boost from any of these products. If you believe a few shots of Body Ammo will make you run farther, longer and stronger, then it probably will—but only because you *think* it will. Once you grasp, deep down, that the one real source of energy is yourself, you'll have taken a major step forward in the struggle to be the best athlete you can be.

DRINK TWO GLASSES OF WATER BEFORE YOU RUN

A runner needs plenty of water before, during and after a run, or there may be problems. Dehydration is the hidden enemy of runners. So if you want to be a runner, become a drinker. Drink at least two glasses of water before you start to run, and if it's to be anything over 6 miles, drink enough water beforehand to make you urinate. Then you know you're hydrated. You shouldn't depend on a feeling of dryness or thirst to tell you when you need a drink of water during a race. By the time you feel thirsty, you'll already be in trouble.

Endurance events demand a lot of energy from your body, and to meet those demands your body needs water. If you don't supply it, if you don't replace the water you lose through sweating, your body can't work efficiently. It could break down completely. You may become dizzy or nauseated, or you may collapse from overheating. You could die. So in a big race, you ought to drink 6 or 8 ounces, or more, at regular intervals. Don't skip the water stations just to be macho or shave off a few seconds from your running time.

What you drink isn't important, so long as you're taking in fluid. All those fancy electrolyte concoctions may make you feel great as you swill them down, but your body will do just as well with good old plain water. If Mother Nature had wanted you to drink Gatorade, she'd have made you sweat Gatorade. A good diet will give you all the salt and electrolytes you need; in fact, the chances are that your diet already has too much salt in it. Runners should not take salt tablets; that extra salt only adds to the risk of dehydration. To keep going, what you need is water.

COPING WITH BOREDOM

Some runners have to battle weak knees and others have to cope with sore feet and blisters, but there's not a runner alive who hasn't had to deal with boredom. We're not used to spending long periods of time alone, with ourselves, quiet time, time to think or not think, time to be whoever we want to be and feel whatever we want to feel. Some runners adore the opportunity; others find it a real burden, but most probably waver back and forth between good days and bad days, easy days when the 5 miles flew by and tough days when 5 miles seemed to take 5 hours.

There are things you can do to fight boredom, tricks you can play with your body, on your mind. They won't always work but they'll keep you busy trying, and that alone is sometimes enough to break through the boredom barrier. One thing you can try is to alter your running speed and rhythm. The running Spinos, Mike and Dyveke—once both instrumental in the Esalen Sports Center, now divorced and running their lives on separate tracks—are very big on teaching recreational runners to alternate slow runs with fast sprints, to run 100 yards emphasizing the left leg lift and then 100 yards emphasizing the right, even to flip around and run sidewards or backward if the mood strikes and the path is clear.

They like their runners to spice up their running with relaxation techniques before and after, and like many teachers in the growing body consciousness field, they teach runners to use visualization to keep the mind from thinking it's bored. One such visualization involves running along and imagining a huge hand pushing you along from behind. Or spotting a tree 80 yards or more ahead, and imagining yourself being reeled in, effortlessly, toward that tree. The imagined pull becomes irresistible and next thing you know you're 20 yards past the tree and all your thoughts of quitting for the day have been cleverly waylaid. Which is another way of saying, use your imagination when you run. Notice the trees, the birds, the clouds, the smells. Count squirrels or cars or footfalls. See how many other runners you can get to wave back.

Have you ever tried to run with your eyes closed? Blind runners do it all the time but it sure is scary. Try it with a friend running alongside one day, just to see how it feels. There are dozens of tricks you can try and, in Marilynn's mind, we may have saved the best one for last. She runs with a set of AM-FM headphones, sometimes tuned to classical music, most often to an early morning replay of a 90-minute award-winning national public radio news show called "All Things Considered." The purists will say that's cheating, but it sure beats boredom. And most important of all, it keeps her going.

If you want to pursue the subject, there are books that deal with it at length—Dyveke Spino's *New Age Training for Fitness and Health* (Grove Press, 1979) and George Sheehan's *Running and Being* are two of them.

WOMEN AND RUNNING

CAN I RUN IF I'M PREGNANT?

Women ask us this question all the time. The answer is yes. Women runners who get pregnant can most likely continue to run and not have to worry about damaging the fetus. There are a few extra risks that should be considered: swollen ankles may make you more susceptible to sprains; ligaments in the pelvic area may stretch and tear more easily. But if you're diligent about warm-ups and careful not to overdo, there's no good reason to quit. Indeed, mothers-to-be who are fit and stay in condition throughout their pregnancy have a real advantage over those with weak muscle tone and poor circulation. Athletic women tend to have quicker deliveries, less pain and shorter convalescences than nonathletic ones. And they have less lower back pain and faster postpartum recoveries as well, says Dr. Dorothy Harris, director of the Center for Women and Sport at Penn State.

The fetus is well protected inside the uterus, and there is no evidence that once it is firmly implanted, running will jar it loose. However, what is thought to be generally true may not be true for you. If you feel too uncomfortable while you're running. or if you develop pain, bleeding or any other symptom that seems out of the ordinary, you should stop running and see your doctor.

WHAT'S THE BEST BRA TO WEAR?

Women who run, pregnant or not, should wear something to support their breasts if their breasts are big enough to bounce and hurt.

Several name-brand manufacturers have come up with special designs for women athletes who need to keep breast tissue from tearing, but don't want the bra to rub or poke or dig into the shoulders. You'll have to shop around until you find a style to suit you; in the meantime you can improvise with a 6-inch elastic bandage, wrapped securely but not tight enough to leave marks. It's not the most glamorous way to go, but it's inexpensive and works.

WHAT ABOUT FLAB?

Women who run are frequently concerned about their figures. If you stick to a program of regular running, and don't eat any more than before, you will lose weight. It may not happen as fast as you might like (because fat turns into muscle and muscle weighs more), but you will undoubtedly lose inches, firm up your trunk and legs and come down a dress size or two. One thing running won't do is eliminate flab. If you've got loose skin where fat used to be, you've got a problem that can only be solved by a plastic surgeon, provided you're willing to go to the trouble and expense. You can turn fat to muscle, and you can make your muscles trimmer, but you can't run off flab. Sorry.

RUNNING HOT AND COLD

The hotter it is outside, the more careful you have to be about drinking plenty of water, and not pushing yourself too hard. If you're very obese and out of condition, you're probably better off sitting out the hottest times of the day. If you're a conditioned athlete, used to running and attentive to signs of overheating—headache, dizziness, nausea and so on—then you can run as far as common sense allows. To help matters, wear clothes that allow sweat to evaporate freely.

When it's bitter cold outside and there's a freezing wind, you may not feel much like running. But from a physiological point of view there's really no danger. The cold air can't freeze your lungs, though it can make you feel uncomfortable at first—especially if you're not in condition. Ice and snow can also make running slippery and treacherous underfoot, so be careful where you step.

Winter is not the best time for a new runner to begin. Even if you've been running, cold weather calls for special precautions. Dress warmly, in layers, keeping in mind how toasty warm you're going to feel when you're 15 minutes into your run; and don't overdo it. Gloves will help you feel comfortable, and so might a face mask. A hat is a real must; it will help retain as much as 50 percent of your body heat. Be sure to give yourself an especially good warm-up when it's cold outside; and afterward, get into warm, dry clothes as soon as possible after you cool down.

10. Swimming

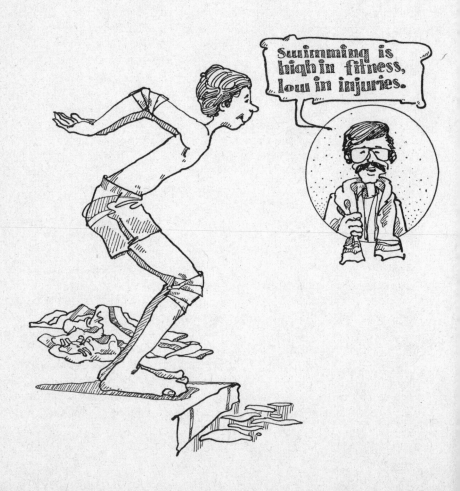

Dear Dr. Jock:

I am 9 years old. Whenever my family goes to the beach or to the pool near where I live, my mom always tells me I should wait at least 30 minutes after I eat to go in swimming. Otherwise, she says, I will get a cramp. My question is why would I get a cramp in the water from eating a hot dog if I don't get a cramp when I eat it somewhere else, like at home? Thank you.

B.C., Gainesville, Florida

Dear Dr. Jock:

I'm on the girls' swim team in my school and my problem is I don't have a lot of strength in my upper arms. The coach says I should work with weights. What should I do? Is it dangerous? I don't want to end up looking like a boy!

S.F., Los Angeles, California

Dear Dr. Jock:

We just moved into a modern high-rise building with a great big indoor pool. I started to swim laps and in 3½ weeks have worked myself up to 35 (without stopping), but I am getting so bored with it I could scream. What can I do? What can I think about? I don't want to quit but the thought of continuing to be bored is equally dreadful.

D.T., Des Moines, Iowa

Claudia hated swimming. When she was in high school, she used to beg her doctor for a note to get out of it. Or she'd fake an excuse and hope her teacher didn't recall it was the third Thursday that month she was claiming to be—what was the cliché in her high school?—regular.

Claudia hated swimming because she thought it was boring. Up and back, up and back, stroke after stroke, breath after breath, the same thing over and over . . . b-o-r-i-n-g. Besides that, the water was always so cold. And the tank suits were ugly, and the chlorine burned her eyes, and water ruined her hair for the rest of the day.

That was twenty years ago.

Today, Claudia is 35 and she swears that swimming (along with hand-held hair dryers) has saved her life. She got hooked on it when she joined the health club near her job and now she does it regularly 3 or 4 times a week, at least 40 minutes or 75 laps, depending. She's lost 18 pounds, gained two hours of extra energy a day, and for the first time ever, someone at the agency actually told her she had nice legs. She's stopped biting her nails, too, and doesn't tug at her hair any more. Swimming has given her a long, lean look without leaving her hungry, and she hasn't missed a session or a day of work in over fifteen months.

Stan likes swimming for a different set of reasons. His office is only three blocks away from the Y and he can usually manage a half-hour swim either before work, after 6 or at lunch time. He's a high-pressure sales executive, always shuffling a dozen different deals at once, his mind constantly buzzing from one minor crisis to another. That swim is the only time all day when he can slow down and ease up. He uses the time to think out problems, or he may not think at all, except to count off the laps, one by one. Though the first 10 minutes can be a bore, by the end of the half hour he feels refreshed, renewed. He tried running for several years but his knees were giving him so much trouble that he had to stop. Stan says (and his doctor agrees), now that he's been swimming his knees are in better shape than ever before.

SWIMMING IS A TOP CONDITIONER

Chalk up two satisfied customers for swimming, one of the best fitness sports around. It enables you to stretch and strengthen many of the major muscle groups, with the added advantage of having all that water to buoy you up, help you defy gravity and deny stress its terrible toll on your body.

We don't absolutely know what long, slow distance running will do to your joints after fifteen or twenty years, but with swimming that is not a concern. You don't get any of the wear and tear on the knees and ankles, or the elbows, and so on, that you do with running or tennis or soccer.

Swimming is also excellent therapy for any athlete who needs to rehabilitate a knee following surgery. Thanks to the water's buoyancy, it is possible to work muscles and joints that might not otherwise move, and it can be done with relatively little pain. (That's why some arthritis patients do so well when they get started on a regular program of pool exercise.) Even if you can't actually swim, you can get a decent workout just trying a slow run back and forth across the shallow end of the pool. If you think that isn't work, try 15 minutes of running in chest-high water, and watch what happens to your pulse rate.

Swimming is a good cardiovascular conditioner—providing you follow Chapter 3 and do it at least 3 times a week, 30 minutes at a time, and at a fast enough pace to push your pulse to between 60 and 85 percent of your maximal heart rate. It has a low risk of injury as compared to running and cycling. Except for competitive swimmers who practice from 4 to 6 hours a day, or marathon swimmers like Stella Taylor or Diana Nyad, who subject themselves to all manner of physical and mental tortures, few swimmers develop muscle or joint problems. It is true that you can slip and fall on the slippery edge of a pool, or cripple yourself for life if you dive in headfirst at the shallow end—and that in 1977 an estimated 56,400 children and adults ended up in hospital emergency rooms as a result of swimming-pool accidents. A few common-sense rules would go far toward preventing most such injuries: don't let kids swim alone, build a fence around an unsupervised pool, don't horse around, watch where you're diving and so on. Other problems that swimmers encounter—conjunctivitis, swimmer's elbow, athlete's foot—will be treated later on in this chapter.

WARMING UP, SWIMMING STRONGER

Warm-up exercises are less crucial for swimmers than for runners because the smooth, rhythmic strokes are not especially stressful, and seldom lead to muscle pulls. General loosening-up exercises don't hurt, however; see the chart in Chapter 7 for specific suggestions. And after some hard swimming, you shouldn't forget about taking 5 to 10 minutes to cool yourself down and let the body's blood flow return to normal.

Strengthening exercises are becoming more and more important in competitive swimming. In the summer of 1978 the U.S. Women's team swamped the East German one in the World Championship races, and the coaches say that the showing was due at least partly to greater emphasis on working with weights. A swimmer who wants to improve both speed and endurance will find some specific muscle-strengthening advice in the chart on pages 152–153.

Too many people are turned off swimming because of a look at a Mark Spitz or a young Cynthia Woodhead. Knowing they'll never look that good, they give up on the whole idea before they begin. You don't have to be a champion free-styler to soak up all the benefits of slow distance swimming. Get in and start stroking as best you can, on your back, on your side, on your belly—and don't stop until at least 30 minutes are up. Your form will improve in more ways than one if you stick with it, but if you never even have the guts to start, you're really sunk.

SWIMMERS CAN GET TENDINITIS, TOO

Though swimmers are less likely to overuse their muscles than those engaging in more stressful sports such as running, it's still not impossible. Some competitive swimmers develop pain in the shoulders. Usually the trouble is a tendinitis, caused by forcing the shoulder through a greater range of motion than it is used to. Few of us have jobs or lives that require us to lift our hands over our heads, but if you're swimming a crawl, you may do it 50-70 times a minute. Since the muscles aren't flexible enough in that unaccustomed position, important shoulder tendons may be torn just a little—and that can bring on the start of tendinitis. (For the details on this painful subject, see Chapter 4.) Older athletes are especially vulnerable to shoulder tendinitis, because of the tightening that goes with age. Keeping stretched and flexible is the way to prevent this problem. That means doing arm and shoulder stretches before you do your laps—or any time at all, for that matter. While you're waiting for the bus, for instance, lift one hand up over your shoulder and as far down the back as you can, and reach around behind your back with the opposite hand and try to clasp your hands in midback. When you get that position, or as close to it as you can, hold it for a few thoughtful seconds and feel the stretch. Then reverse hands.

A swimmer who already has a tender shoulder needn't worry about having to give up swimming. You may have to work your way around and through the pain, but meanwhile the tendinitis will be healing itself. Try to shorten your stroke as you swim and use ice on your shoulder afterward, to cut down on pain and swelling. If you need further relief, try aspirin 4 times a day. If you're still hurting too much to go on, you'd better see a doctor.

The second problem peculiar to swimmers is even less common. The frog kick, primarily used in the breaststroke, puts a lot of strain on the medial collateral ligament, on the inside of the knee. Constant repetition can sprain the ligament and cause pain that can take the pleasure out of swimming—though it usually doesn't interfere with walking. The only way to prevent the problem is building up strength and flexibility by conditioning yourself gradually. Meanwhile, switch from the breaststroke to a crawl or sidestroke when you swim, and it will eventually go away.

SWIMMING CAN BE INFECTIOUS

A swimming pool can be a very relaxing, mind-cleansing environment. It can also be the breeding ground for several little bugs, with big Latin names (*Pseudomonas aeruginosa* and *Mycobacterium balnei,* etc.) that are capable of producing blotches, itching and pain. Haphazard maintenance and inadequate chlorination turn a pool into an infectious soup. On the other hand, too much chlorine can also be annoying (wear goggles), so you have to hope for (and be responsible for) striking some happy balance.

Don't swim if you've got a runny nose or open sores, and encourage others not to. Swimming pool elbow—a tender red bump that develops into a crusted ulcer after you've bumped or scraped your elbow in an infected pool—can be a serious problem. If it doesn't heal in a reasonable time, you should see a dermatologist. Be sure to mention that you're a regular swimmer, since that will help in the diagnosis.

SWIMMERS' EAR

Another problem you might run into if you swim regularly is an infection of the ear canal, medically known as otitis externa. It's usually caused by *Pseudomonas* bacteria, and a major symptom is itching. There is seldom much pain. Some people seem to be more susceptible to this than others and it can occur in a properly chlorinated pool. Ask your doctor to give you a prescription for ear drops, or try an over-the-counter remedy.

CONJUNCTIVITIS

If you've been swimming, and all of a sudden your eyes get red, itchy and hot, a virus or a bacterial infection picked up in the pool is probably the cause. The official name of the disease is conjunctivitis, and what happens is that the mucous membrane that lines the eyelid and covers your eyeball becomes inflamed. It is generally painful enough so that you won't have to think twice before calling the doctor. In the meantime, a loose eyepatch will help make it feel better, but be careful about using cotton—it could dry up the eye and make the pain even worse. Your doctor will probably give you an antibiotic to help clear up the inflammation. In the meantime, you don't *have* to quit swimming for your own sake, but you should consider the other people who use the pool. If you've picked up a virus, you could be spreading it. Better stay clear of the pool until the inflammation is gone.

ATHLETE'S FOOT

This is a fungus that is usually picked up in public places. It settles in areas that are warm and moist, such as between your toes. Swimmers get it mainly from hanging around wet locker rooms and pool areas. The best prevention of the disease—known medically as tinea pedis—is to keep your feet as dry as possible. Drying and powdering them thoroughly *after* swimming should be standard practice. If you do get the bug, and your feet are itchy and red, you might try a commercial remedy first. If that doesn't help, see a doctor. Athlete's foot can be cured; but once you've gotten it, it's likely to come back time and time again.

STOMACH CRAMPS—PANIC CAN KILL YOU

Mention swimming and safety to almost anyone, child or adult, and one of the first things you can expect to hear is that you should wait at least a half hour after eating before you swim. It's one of the oldest clichés of sports medicine—and it's perfectly true. If you've had any sort of meal at all (a hot dog and soft drink qualifies; a popsicle doesn't), serious cramps really can set in if you swim too soon afterward. The cramps themselves aren't so serious, but the panic they may cause is another thing altogether. What happens too often is that instead of shouting a few times for help and then going to work on calming yourself and getting rid of the cramp, you go on yelling, bouncing up and down and taking in too much water. Under those conditions, it is frighteningly easy to drown.

Why do you cramp in the first place? That is a good question, because knowing the answer goes a long way toward making sure you won't drown. You get a cramp because some working muscle—usually one in your leg—is not getting enough oxygen to perform properly, and it goes into a spasm. And the reason it's not getting enough oxygen is because your blood supply has been diverted to your stomach to help digest your meal. What you need to get rid of the cramp is more oxygen in your system, so that you can handle *both activities*. The way to take in more oxygen is a long series of deep breaths. If you concentrate on that instead of on the cramp, you have a good chance of coming out of the crisis alive.

WHAT TO DO ABOUT BOREDOM

Swimming can be a bore, but no more so than running—and more than 25 million people are managing to lick that problem; as a swimmer you can do the same. Do what the runners do—play little mind games with yourself. If you've got a problem at work or at home or with a friend, the perfect time to think about it is while you're swimming. If your mind is already buzzing with too much brain noise, now's the time to calm down. Concentrate on your breathing (belly out when you inhale, belly in when you exhale) and get it going at a rhythm that suits you. You have an advantage over runners in that there are no distractions from the outside world. You can think about whatever you choose, or you can choose not to think at all. You can use the counting ploy—mentally drawing each number as you say it, or visualizing yourself building each number out of mortar and brick (one lap equals one number; when you're finished with 100 laps, you have a row of well-built numbers stretching halfway down the block). If you get tired of that, watch the pattern of light as it dances across the bottom of the pool. Or start a mental list of all the sounds you can hear.

Do whatever you have to do, but keep going. It will help to vary your strokes, and vary your pace. A respectable overhand crawl, by the way, will burn up about 9 calories per minute, as compared with 8 for the backstroke and something under 7 calories per minute for the breaststroke. The butterfly stroke is the most demanding, and uses up 12 calories per minute. To achieve a training effect, as we've said, you should be swimming fast enough to push your pulse to between 60 and 85 percent of your maximal rate. More important to your overall program is not how fast or how hard you swim, but how often and for how long a stretch—at least 3 times a week, for 30 minutes at a time. If you go slower, swim longer.

Unless you've learned to swim recently, you probably were taught the crawl the old way—to pull your arm up out of the water, keeping it close to your ear, and throw it forward with your hand slightly cupped as you cut into the water. A newer version of the crawl stroke is not only easier and more efficient, but also less stressful to your arm. To do it, keep your elbow bent slightly as you swim. As you bring your arm out of the water, think about entering it again at a point along the midline of your body. Let your hand enter the water as though you were slipping a letter into one of those trapdoor mailboxes. Then, keeping your elbow comfortably bent, pull your whole arm down toward your crotch. To Marilynn, this seems a much more natural, less tiring stroke than the old-style crawl—so much easier that it's almost like cheating.

Marilynn also cheats (sort of) as she swims her mile, by wearing a scuba mask and snorkel. It looks a little weird in an indoor pool, but it keeps her going and solves the problem she was having with the coordination of breathing and stroking. Using the snorkel, she can keep her breathing nice and steady and her strokes long and hard, and doesn't have to worry about lifting and twisting her head out of the water with every other beat. What's nice about swimming with your head under water is the mesmerizing peace and quiet you feel. It's easier to concentrate, easier to get lost, and the effort is pleasant when you're certain you won't be swallowing more water than you're comfortable with. Using a mask and snorkel is just another way of finding *your* way to keep going. If you think it'll hook you on regular swimming, try it. We don't recommend fins, however—that really *would* be cheating.

11. Cycling

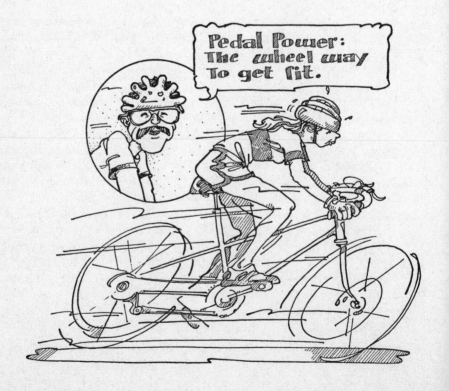

Dear Dr. Jock:

I bought a 10-speed last summer, and this year, for the first time, I've started to do some serious riding. I'm 25, live and work in the city, and I find if I ride for an hour really early in the morning, before work and before traffic, it does me a world of good. My problem sounds silly but it's serious to me: I am getting such a sore butt I can barely stand to continue riding. In fact, sometimes I have to stand! Is there anything I can do about this?

F.P., Atlanta, Georgia

Dear Dr. Jock:

My friend and I are 16 years old and we've been saving up and making plans to ride the Bikecentennial trail across country next year. Can you tell us what we should do to get ready for it? We thought maybe we'd lift weights but we're not sure. Any tips? (My friend says to ask you what we should carry in our first-aid kit, too.)

L.H., Easton, Pennsylvania

Dear Dr. Jock:

Can a person get fit riding a stationary bike? I am tempted to buy one but before I do I want to know what good it will do me, if any. I tried bicycling one other time and I liked it but I kept getting a lot of pain in my right knee and I had to quit. Now I'm a widow, 64, and I feel I have to do something with myself or I'll just go to pieces. What about those exercycles?

I.K., Skokie, Illinois

The big bicycle boom of the early 1970s may be over, but cycling as a leisure-time activity keeps rolling on. A recent government survey ranked it as the second favorite recreational sport in the country, right behind walking. More than 100 million Americans ride bikes, and between 1972 and 1976 bicycles actually outsold cars by nearly 10 million units. The statistics show the average cyclist in this country to be 34 years old. (We guessed 11½.) He or she rides the bike an average of 3 times a week for 9 months of the year, and averages an impressive 2,300 miles a year.

And why shouldn't they? A bike is easy to buy, cheap to run, and if you ride it regularly, you're almost sure to start feeling better than you've felt in a long time. Like tennis or softball or golf, cycling is fun and it can be a delightful way for an entire family to spend a sunny Sunday afternoon. But ahead of tennis, softball and especially golf, bicycling ranks among the Big Three as a conditioner—with running and swimming. It's not as safe a sport as swimming, but it causes far fewer foot, knee and leg problems than running. Like running, it won't do much to beef up your biceps or reduce flabby arms. However, a properly designed fitness program that revolves around cycling will do wonders for your cardiovascular system. If you use your bicycle at least 3 times a week, and if you do it at a rhythmical, steady speed for at least 30 minutes at a time—not to be confused with a 5-minute dash to the corner store—at a speed and pace of sufficient intensity to challenge your body and make your heart work, then you are on the road to fitness.

PEDAL YOUR PRESSURES AWAY

Long-distance cyclists frequently talk about their sport in the same passionate language runners use. Once they're into their rhythm, into themselves, man and mind and machine are one: spirits lift, energy soars and the petty aggravations of life somehow get lost in the endless spinning of the wheels. A bicycle can carry you somewhere you want to remember, or it can whisk you away from a place you'd rather forget; you're the rider, you determine the route. An hour's brisk bicycle ride through the city or a park or down a country road in the early morning, before the traffic, can be a great way to clear the morning cobwebs, calm the working fears and begin a beautiful day. For many people, cycling is a welcome escape away from pressures and problems and toward something healthy, positive, pleasurable. A bicycle is an especially cheap, efficient way to travel, too, from home to office, from city to city, from inn to inn, from country to country . . . and one day, when you feel up to something like 2 million pedal strokes, you may want to join the hardy breed of cross-country cyclists who are keeping the Bikecentennial spirit alive. It's a trip of 4,500 miles from Reedsport, Oregon, to Yorktown, Virginia, and bicyclists of greatly varying ages, backgrounds, ability and experience take part. Indeed, Drs. Daniel Kulund and Clifford Brubaker surveyed 89 Bikecentennial riders (64 men, from 17 to 66 years old; 25 women, from 17 to 54 years old) and concluded that bike touring is a safe and desirable activity that presents only the most modest medical problems to healthy cyclists, even untrained ones.

Don't be misled, however. Yes, bicycling is good for you, and there is a fairly low risk of bringing on a sports-related ailment. But there is a grimmer side to the picture. An estimated one million accidents and almost a thousand deaths each year are associated with bicyclists, according to the U.S. Consumer Product Safety Commission. A bicycle is not a toy; it's a vehicle, and the Commission has it listed as the country's single most hazardous product.

YOUR SAFETY DEPENDS ON YOU

Educating yourself to be the best bicyclist you can be will unquestionably cut the risk of accident. Accidents frequently involve losing control of the bike. You hit a bump, you misjudge a curb or a turn, or you let yourself get flustered by traffic. Being comfortable in traffic takes time and training. Most of the collisions between cyclists and drivers are due to the cyclist's negligence—running through a stop sign, traveling the wrong way down a street or, most frequently, darting in and out of traffic as though there were absolutely nothing to fear from a 3,000-pound, motor-driven, gas-burning competitor.

So, even though it sounds like kid stuff, brush up on biking safety. Learn the rules of the road. Don't ride the wrong way down a one-way street. Don't ride at night if you can't see or be seen. Signal turns, especially left turns. To be seen more easily, wear light-colored and/or reflective clothing and make sure your bike is properly outfitted with lights and safety reflectors. Sometimes, one of those big Day-Glo-colored flags attached to the back of a bicycle will help draw attention and repel absentminded drivers.

Above all, be alert and aware of what you are doing and where you are going on your bike. If you're tooling down a country highway at a steady clip and there's no traffic, only miles of uninterrupted blacktop, you can afford to let your attention dwell on what a lovely day it is, and how much better the countryside looks, smells, even tastes when you're not seeing it from behind the bug-splattered windshield of an air-conditioned auto. Those are the best times of bicycling, when it's you and the bike and the open road. But when you're in the city, you should practice more defensive driving. You have to be acutely aware of traffic, pedestrians, potholes, glass, sewer bumps and a dozen other hazards if you want to stay out of trouble.

KNOW YOUR BIKE AND HOW IT WORKS

The second most important way to stay injury-and-trouble-free is to take proper care of your bicycle. Structural or mechanical problems can involve you in a nasty accident when you least expect it. So buy a book, take a course, see your local shop owner or do whatever you have to do to learn the basics of bicycle maintenance and repair.

And finally, to make the most of your bicycling and the least of your problems, learn the most practical and efficient way to bicycle. A 1-speed or a 3-speed bicycle may be perfectly adequate for 10-mile trips with the family or a run to the corner for a carton of milk; but if you plan to ride your bike long enough and hard enough to boost fitness, you'll do well to invest in a 10-speed bike. The light frame, low-slung handlebars, narrow seat and bent-over riding position of a 10-speed bike may seem awkward at first, but in fact it's the most practical way to go. Though 10 gears may seem like too much to cope with at first, don't slide into the habit of sticking with one gear. Learn when and why to shift. It'll make your bicycling easier, not harder, especially going uphill, and it will help you maintain an even tempo or cadence.

Experts say a beginning rider should be able to maintain a consistent 45 revolutions per minute (rpm), whereas some top cyclists may reach 100 rpm. Go at your own pace, but keep going and build your endurance, duration and intensity gradually.

PROBLEMS AND DISCOMFORTS

The warm-up for riding is no problem at all. You just start out your ride slowly, noticing any spots of tightness or tension. The more you bicycle, the better your condition, the less likely you are to develop any kind of medical difficulty. Problems will arise, however, from time to time, especially if the course you've set for yourself involves strenuous hill-climbing. Naturally, the more you know about the problems you might encounter—their causes and treatment—the easier it will be for you to avoid them.

SEAT DISCOMFORT

This is one of the most common and least serious complaints among beginning bicyclists. Those hard, narrow racing seats do take some getting used to, but they are much better for you over the long haul than the wider, softer seats. Try different sizes, different brands, until you find the best seat for you and ask your local bike shop owner for some help.

If you're getting a lot of rubbing, chafing and pain, check your shorts. Heavy seams and a too-tight fit can be quite irritating. Look for shorts that are soft and comfortable. Special jersey and chamois cycling shorts are made without seams in the crotch to help reduce friction. Baby or talcum powder sprinkled in and around your shorts will do the same. No matter how sore you feel, don't use liniment and heat products like Ben Gay on that area. After a while, if you stick to your riding, your butt will toughen up and the discomfort will go away.

For men, there's another sort of seat pain that can be alarming. It's called ischemic neuropathy of the penis—a numbness that can occur after cycling 40 or more miles a day at a steady pace, as a result of prolonged pressure. The numbness may last from a few minutes to two days. You shouldn't continue riding until you get the feeling back. If you don't get it back in a couple of days, you should see a doctor.

KNEE PAIN

Another common problem with cyclists is often a result of trying too much, too soon. There's no reason to avoid hills when you're cycling, but they do require you to work harder and they can put extra stress on the patellar tendons. Too much extra stress can cause considerable pain, though this usually subsides when you stop cycling. Like the tendinitis associated with running, it is best prevented by gradual conditioning.

Sometimes you can bring on unnecessary knee pain by riding your bicycle with the seat set at an improper height. Check it yourself or see the smartest mechanic at your local bike shop. Your leg should be about 90 percent extended when your pedal is at the bottom of your downstroke. You can set the position by sitting on the bicycle and placing your heel on the pedal with your knee straight. Then, with the seat adjusted to that height, when you ride with your toes and the ball of the foot on the pedal, it should be just about right. If the height's right and you're still feeling pain, try readjusting the seat until your knee finds some relief. Don't be afraid to experiment. The idea with any sort of tendinitis is to get rid of the pain—the condition will heal itself in time. You don't have to quit riding but you do have to deal with the pain.

There are several things you can try on your own to relieve pain around the knee. Some riders use liniment, or they ride in long pants so the tendon can warm up and stretch out more. Riding with an elastic bandage may or may not help. If you use one, be sure not to wrap it too tight. You can also try body awareness and visualization techniques for relaxing your muscles and increasing your sense of flow; more details about this are given in Chapter 5. The more you relax, the more steady you feel, the more confident you get, the easier it'll be for you to ride through your pain and enjoy the afternoon.

If the pain is still there after you stop cycling, use an ice pack for 20 or 30 minutes, 3 or 4 times every 24 hours if necessary.

HAND PAIN

Long-distance cycling can be a pain in the hand, too. In the traditional tripod position of the easy rider, the hands bear a lot of pressure and sometimes the fleshy part of the heel of the hand, or the base of the inner hand away from the thumb, begins to hurt. Naturally, gradual conditioning will toughen the hand. Padded handlebars, tape and riding gloves will help, too. You can also try switching riding positions. Rough, bumpy roads aggravate the situation. Riding with no hands may bring immediate relief, followed by major disaster. Don't do it.

You really don't have to worry about hand pain unless it's accompanied by numbness. Your ulnar nerve runs through a tight canal, and when too much pressure is applied for too long, the nerve can be injured. If it is, you'll be numb in the little finger and, usually, in part of the ring finger. You may also experience some weakness, and have trouble getting your fingers to work properly. If you can't relieve the numbness and loss of motion by padding the handlebars and wearing gloves, then you ought to quit riding and give the nerve a chance to recover. If your hand is still numb and weak the next day, you should not continue riding until the symptoms disappear. And if they don't disappear in a few days, see a doctor.

There's another nerve, the median, that you have to watch out for. It crosses the wrist at the middle of the palmar surface and it too is enclosed in a tight canal. Prolonged pressure on it can cause numbness in the thumb, the index and middle fingers, and part of the ring finger. This is called carpal tunnel syndrome, and you should treat it with the same caution as you do trouble with the ulnar nerve. Neither of these hand problems should be ridden through or toughed out. They can be serious, and may result in permanent injury.

ANKLE PAIN

Achilles tendinitis is not uncommon in cyclists. The symptoms are similar to those that runners get: pain with ankle motion, tenderness over the tendon, some swelling and redness. This problem occurs because of poor conditioning. It's an overuse syndrome belonging to the "too much, too soon" category of physical unfitness. Ankling is a good technique to know for riding, but doing it too vigorously may overstress the Achilles tendon and bring on a tendinitis. If you are having a problem, adjusting the seat should help.

Another source of ankle pain is improper shoes. Special cycling shoes with a metal clamp on the sole may help make your pedaling easier, though they are not a must-have as running shoes are for runners. However, shoes that come up too high on the back of the ankle may cause pain by rubbing the Achilles tendon.

To treat your tendinitis, apply ice to the painful area after you ride. It is all right to ride as long as you can stand the pain.

BACK PAIN

It's a funny thing about back pain and bicycling. Some riders believe cycling causes it; others find that a nice long run, stretched and balanced over a 10-speed bike, can actually relieve a tense, painful back. Bicycling can bring on back pain if you're tense and fearful when you ride. Stretching out over low-slung handlebars may make you feel awkward and vulnerable at first, but the sooner you learn to relax and ease the tensions in your back, neck and shoulders, the better off you'll be.

When you ride in the tripod position, keep the weight evenly balanced on your feet, your seat and your hands. Keeping the abdominal muscles strong and tight will reduce strain on the back and the best way to do that is with bent-knee sit-ups. If you have a bad back already, and you're looking for a good sport, swimming would be your best bet but bicycling is worth a try. If you experience too much pain riding, rest until the pain subsides, and try to build up your endurance slowly and gradually with sit-ups followed by slow cycling.

STATIONARY CYCLES AS CONDITIONERS

Finally, a word about the relative merits of getting your exercise on a stationary bike. The word is yes, you can put together a perfectly adequate fitness regimen for yourself using a stationary bike, as long as you use it in a way that satisfies the three requirements of frequency, intensity and duration. But *you* have to do the work. Having one of those motor-driven exercycles push and pull your feet through the motions of pedaling won't do you much good.

Choose a stationary bike that is strong and steady enough to support you in motion, and make sure it has a tension control adjustment so you can continue to challenge yourself as you get stronger. Begin slowly, so as to warm and stretch your muscles, and when the ride is over, slow down and cool down so you won't be bothered with aches and pains. Adjust the seat so that you can get the proper 90 percent leg extension on your downstroke.

The advantage of a stationary bike is that you can get your exercise at home, any time of day, maybe even in front of the evening news, or listening to Brahms on the stereo. The disadvantage is that you encounter nothing and no one you haven't seen before. You don't get the smells of freshly cut grass, of summer leaving and leaves turning. It's as different from real riding as jogging on a treadmill is from a glorious morning run along the beach. But if it's your way, your choice and it keeps you going, that's what matters.

12. Skiing

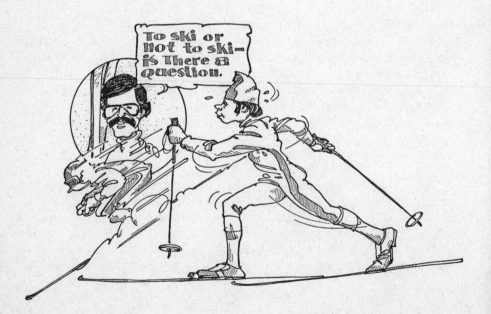

Dear Dr. Jock:

Last time my husband and I went skiing (one week at Snowbird in Utah), I came down with a bad case of the high altitude blues. I had a headache for two days straight and no energy whatsoever. What causes this and what can I do about it next time (if there is a next time!)?

J.L., Buffalo, New York

Dear Dr. Jock:

Can you give me a program I can follow to get ready for the cross-country ski season? I took up the sport last year and really liked it. It was the most fun I've ever had in winter and this year is the first time since I was a small child that I'm actually looking forward to heavy snow. But I haven't done any sports all year and my whole body feels like wet cement. What can I do?

B.P., Chicago, Illinois

Dear Dr. Jock:

My friend is a cross-country skier and I am strictly a downhiller. We've taken several ski vacations together but he always goes his way and I go mine. Now we're wondering which sport is better for fitness. I think mine because it's faster but he says cross-country. Who's right?

R.R., San Francisco, California

Winter used to be something we had to survive. Skiing has made it something to look forward to. It doesn't matter whether you do downhill or cross-country, skiing is one of the most popular and thrilling sports you can do. *If* you do it reasonably well. And *if* you do it reasonably safely.

You can be a lousy tennis player and not do yourself much damage, and you can be a pretty reckless runner and not get into too much trouble if you just stay on track. But if you don't know what you're

189

doing and you wind up doing it on skis, headed down a mountain at 30 miles an hour, you're probably going to wind up in a heap of trouble and tangled limbs. So our first word of advice about skiing is to learn the sport. Take lessons, join a group, read books, learn from a pal, watch TV, do whatever you have to do to master the basics first.

GETTING READY FOR THE SKI SEASON

Skiing is a seasonal sport. So unless you're keeping up your fitness throughout the year, it's likely that many muscles you need to be strong and flexible are, in fact, weak and tight. So the first thing you need is a strength-and-flexibility program. You'll find the information you need about this in Chapters 7 and 8.

It would be best to start your program anywhere from six to eight weeks before your first ski trip. During this time, swear off elevators and take the stairs every chance you get. Walking up steps—two at a time is best—and walking down them too, is a terrific way to build strength in your leg muscles.

Another good body builder is jumping rope. Not only will it build your endurance and lessen fatigue on the slopes, but it will also increase your agility. Skipping rope only looks like kid stuff. Try doing it at a steady rapid rate and you'll see why it's such a good all-over body conditioner. An adult will need to use an adult-size jump rope, preferably one with weighted handles that give a comfortable grip. To find the right length, put both feet on the middle of the rope and make sure that the handles reach your armpits. When you jump, wear a good, solidly cushioned pair of athletic shoes—running shoes are fine. Socks cut down friction and help prevent blisters. Don't jump on the bare floor if you can avoid it. Landing hard on the balls of your feet many times can hurt them. If you can jump at all (and it may take some practice on your part to get the skipping part down pat), be sure not to overdo it. You might want to alternate jumping for 10 or 15 seconds with resting for the same length of time. Build up your jumping time gradually. Do stretching warm-ups (especially for the shoulders and calves) before you jump, and cool down gradually afterward. Working out every other day will give tender feet a chance to recover and will cut down on any soreness.

In skiing, unlike some other sports, brute strength isn't nearly as important as agility, balance and flexibility, so whatever exercises you choose should develop those particular abilities. You'll want to concentrate on your leg muscles. Both the quadriceps and the hamstring muscles have to be strong if you are going to be able to control your skis. Cross-country skiing uses the calf muscles more than most sports, and you should give them extra time and attention in warm-ups beforehand. Don't forget arm strength and flexibility either. In cross-country skiing, your arm stroke is a crucial part of your overall glide pattern, and you need strength to plant and push those poles properly. For downhill skiers who spend long periods of time in a bent-knee, half-sitting position, the 90-90 wall sit (described in Chapter 8) is a must.

PREVENTING INJURIES

We can't know exactly how many ski injuries there are every year, though we're told that in one recent year the cost of ski injuries in the United States came to an estimated $12 million. If you're young and an infrequent or inexperienced skier, you're likely to hurt yourself skiing downhill unless you know just what you're doing. In cross-country, it's exactly the opposite: the more experienced you are, the more risks you're likely to take. If you have a tendency to ski out of control, either because you're overconfident or because you don't know any better, then you are adding to the risk of injury. It's nice to press your limits when you're on skis, but if you push too hard you can propel yourself right into the hospital. You should study your body equipment and know your limits. While you should always be striving to develop your potential, you shouldn't stretch so far there's no coming back. Everything that goes up in a ski lift must come down and if you're too weary and out of shape to make the return trip, don't start out.

Skiing is hard work, and demands high energy—especially cross-country skiing. The more fit you are physically, the more efficient your cardiovascular system, the more muscle strength and endurance you develop, the more likely you'll be able to meet all the demands of skiing without becoming too fatigued. When you get tired, you fall, and when you fall in skiing, bad things can happen. Your fancy fiberglass ski becomes an efficient lever that can stress and snap your tibia. Or the force may rip into your knee ligaments; a partial tear means pain and swelling, and a complete tear means surgery. Falling and trying to brace yourself can break a clavicle or dislocate a shoulder, and if you hang onto your ski pole too long, you can tear the ligaments on the inside of the base of your thumb. (This injury is called gamekeeper's thumb because old-time gamekeepers used to tear the same ligament when they yanked off the head of a bird or small mammal.) David's wife June managed to do this on her first cross-country ski trip—six miles out! It hurt, and swelled quickly, and she had a cast on it for four weeks, She eventually got back to cross-country, but she doesn't hold on to the poles nearly as tightly any more—which is exactly the advice ski instructors give. That's another good reason to take the time to really learn the sport. Understanding proper ski technique (including how to fall, how to stand up and, most important, how to slow down and stop) is one very important way you can protect yourself against injuries.

Sixty percent of all ski injuries affect the legs. Thirty percent are either knee ligament injuries or tibial fractures. The ski boots people used to wear could snap an ankle when a skier twisted and fell. The new, higher ones available now protect your ankles and allow you better control. The only problem is that they can also be the cause of more serious injuries. When you wear the new kind of boot, if you fall and your binding doesn't release, your leg is subjected to a high, twisting stress that may well take your knee or tibia with it. Ski manufacturers are forever trying to come up with improved ski-and-boot-release combinations, but it is proving to be a very tricky business. One study estimates that 45 percent of all ski injuries occur because of ski bindings that don't release. There is no absolutely safe ski binding—just some that are less safe than others. To protect yourself, don't skimp on bindings. Buy the best pair you can and spend some time, with the manufacturers' literature, or the salesperson, or with your ski instructor, making sure you understand how they work and how to adjust them for proper release. Most skiers have their bindings set too tightly. Be certain yours aren't, and that they are adequately lubricated, mounted and set.

STAYING HAPPY ON THE SLOPES

In skiing, as in all other sports, your body works best when it is neither too hot nor too cold. You may use a lot of energy and work up a sweat skiing downhill, but you can get terribly chilled in between runs. Skiing cross-country, you may be quite cold when you start out; but as you continue the trek, and your body temperature continues to rise, you'll need less and less in the way of clothes to feel comfortable. The solution in both instances is to wear several layers of clothes. The layers will keep you insulated against the cold, and when you feel too warm you can peel off a layer or two. You'll have to experiment to find the combination of wool and/or down or synthetics; but don't neglect the most efficient outer layer of all—a hat. If you keep the top of your head covered when you ski, you'll retain at least 50 percent of the heat (i.e., energy) you're generating. If you are trekking cross-country and sweating hard, take *off* your hat and gloves and see how quickly you cool down. To help regulate your body temperature and reduce fatigue during a cross-country run, you should also drink plenty of water, not just when you feel thirsty, but at regular intervals.

If you take a half day to cross-country ski out into the woods six miles, remember that it's six slow, sometimes painful miles back. If you *know* you're not up to it, don't push yourself. If you *think* you might be up to it, be as aware as you can of your body signals and proceed with caution. Make sure you keep your energy supply up. And take things easy. Just as in running and walking and swimming, in cross-country skiing you're probably better off going for a longer distance at a slower pace than skiing hard and burning out fast.

If at any time your fingers and toes (or your ears or nose) get red and numb and you fear frostbite, do whatever you can to keep those body parts moving and warm. It's important that you have enough room in your boots to wiggle your toes; the more wiggling you do, the more blood keeps circulating and the less likely you are to get frostbite. For your fingers' sake, remember that mittens tend to be warmer than gloves and a combination of the two may be ideal.

At the opposite extreme, skiers also have to protect themselves against too much sun. The sun can be bright in the mountains, especially in springtime, and its reflection off the white snow only increases the intensity. You can get as sunburned skiing in Sun Valley as you can lying on the beach in Mexico. Protect yourself with therapeutic, not cosmetic, sunglasses and read the labels to find a sunscreen with PABA (para-aminobenzoic acid) that blocks out most of the harmful burning rays.

ALTITUDE SICKNESS

If you're planning a mountain ski vacation, don't think you can fly all morning, ski all afternoon, drink all night and wake up the next day feeling great. When you bring your body to a higher altitude than it is used to, it usually needs time to adjust. It can't get enough oxygen at first, and any liquor you drink acts much quicker. If you're smart and want to avoid the symptoms of altitude sickness—headaches, dizziness, nausea, fatigue—you'll give your body the couple of days it needs to adjust to the higher, thinner air. Some people are affected more than others but you'd be wise to ease into a vigorous ski schedule. And be sure you drink plenty of water, since dehydration makes altitude sickness worse.

DOWNHILL VS. CROSS-COUNTRY

Cross-country is a better conditioning sport than downhill skiing. Downhill racers can really get their hearts thumping and pumping—hard enough to produce a training effect, that's for sure—but don't forget that to develop fitness, you have to be able to sustain this raised pulse for 15 minutes. And how many downhill skiers can afford a ski workout 3 times a week, week after week? Cross-country skiing is a more accessible sport, more like running. If you're in an area with snow, all you have to do is head for the local park or public golf course, slap on the wax and the skis, and take off for an hour of slow, steady, vigorous exercise.

Another advantage cross-country skiing has over downhill as a participatory sport is that it's much easier to learn. It could take you years to master enough downhill techniques to really enjoy a run down a fast slope, but for cross-country you can probably pick up what you need in a few hours and start having fun almost immediately. Cross-country skiing is also a safer sport than downhill, statistically; but make no mistake, either one can hurt you seriously if you're not careful.

In downhill skiing, you can spend a long time getting to the top of the mountain so as to spend as short a time as possible coming down. Frequently the premium is on speed, on superfast decisions, on quick jumps and precision turns. The best downhill skiers do have a rhythm, but it's often a staccato beat. You move so fast you can't really appreciate much of what's around you, whereas in cross-country everything around you becomes part of the experience, part of the thrill. Skiing downhill, you feel incredibly exhilarated; skiing cross-country, a downhill run is part of the exhilaration, but so is marching straight up a hill, or breaking new snow in a forest preserve at 7 o'clock in the morning.

Downhill skiing is a demanding sport, and can offer hair-raising thrills, but don't rely on it to get you into shape. Get in shape *before* you do it—by running, swimming, bicycling or whatever—and you'll have a better time doing it.

More and more downhill skiers are combining the two skills into something called ski mountaineering, which keeps them going, up and down hills, all day long. That way, they can escape the long lines, the expensive lift tickets and the overcrowded craziness that downhill skiers have to contend with in some of the country's choicest spots.

MENTAL PREPARATION IS IMPORTANT TOO

If you're keen on becoming a better skier, a gutsier skier, one who enjoys the sport more and gets injured less, then you must get your mind involved. You must be willing to spend some time dealing with all the fears and tensions and anxieties that can lock your knees, cause you to fall and generally get in the way of a good time.

Up until a few years ago, no one talked very much about the need to condition the mind as well as the body. Ski schools focused on technique, drill, form and very little on consciousness. But skiing is a sport that demands concentration. If your mind wanders or wavers or operates against you in any other way, you're skiing below your potential—whereas when your mind is calm and clear and tuned in to what your body is doing, you'll have a much easier, safer time of it.

At least that's the theory, and it is becoming the subject of books and workshops offering new models for instruction—the Inner Skier, the Centered Skier, the Yoga, Zen and Tao Skiers—all designed to acquaint us with mind tricks and body awareness exercises that were foreign to skiing five years ago. Chapter 5 of this book talks about some of these. For more details, there are at least two books—*Inner Skiing*, by Timothy Gallwey and Bob Kriegel, and *Ski with Yoga: Conditioning for the Mind and Body* by Arne Leuchs and Patricia Skalka— which you might find helpful.

COPING WITH FEAR

What do most skiers fear? Fear itself. Fear leaves us all feeling weak and whipped before we've even begun. Just like stress, however, there is good fear and bad fear, and we're only going to worry about the bad sort of fear that makes our muscles tense and our backs stiffen, and sometimes takes our breath away. This sort of fear leads to fatigue and falling, and the more tired we are, the more we fall down, until the whole cycle gets so vicious and frightening it seems there's no way out.

To ski safely, you must learn to get a grip on fear before fear puts the squeeze on you. Awareness is everything: when you feel the butterflies starting to flutter and your knees are turning to jelly and all you want to do is hide under the chair lift and send out for pizza, that's the time to take a few deep breaths and use some freshly oxygenated common sense. What are you afraid of? Is the slope really too difficult for you or are you seeing it as worse than it really is? What are your alternatives to standing frozen, feeling afraid? What can you do, or say to yourself, to replace the fear with positive, constructive thoughts? The questions are simple but the answers are complex and require as much skill and awareness as a perfect series of parallel turns.

In time you can develop that skill, that awareness, that confidence, but you will probably need help. Again, this is where the right ski instructor can be invaluable. Find one that will help you work through your fears, not by pretending they don't exist, but by helping you understand *why* they exist, and what you can do about them.

TAKING YOUR OWN GOOD TIME

Though fear can be a real crippler when it comes to skiing, so can an unhealthy competitive spirit, a compulsive drive to ski better, faster and farther than anybody else. Be content to learn at your own pace, to ski at your own rhythm. Don't waste your time thinking about the other guy when you should be concentrating on keeping your chin up and your body leaning out into the valley. Don't think about how you'll look when you fall, and don't drain your energy with negative thoughts like; "This is too hard. I'll never learn . . ." If you're in a lesson, or halfway up on the chair lift, and your fears are getting the best of you, take a few minutes and a few deep belly breaths to focus your mind on the momentous task at hand.

VISUALIZING THE PERFECT DESCENT

Next time you go out to ski—cross-country or downhill, doesn't matter—remember to use visualization to get you out of a tough spot, just as some of the pros and Olympic champs do. Say, for instance, you're faced with a tough, treacherous run down an icy slope with a big bump in the middle that you absolutely must avoid. Instead of throwing up your poles in panic and sliding down on your butt, try a little mental exercise. Take a moment to relax and visualize the perfect descent. Start a motion picture of it running in your mind. See yourself starting out slow, in control, turning and twisting in perfect rhythm down the slope, along the path you must take to avoid the bump. Seeing yourself do it, sensing it in your mind's eye, makes doing it easier. Try and see.

Tim Gallwey, in *Inner Skiing,* gives this advice to skiers on how to make a smooth, sweeping run: Imagine the slope as a large, empty canvas, on which every curve you make with your skis is a broad, smooth brushstroke. The trick works for some people; it may work for you.

SKI WITH FEELING

Skiing is done at such high speed that you don't have much time for considered opinions. But you do have time to feel, and the more aware you are of what you're feeling on the way down the slope, the better your skiing will be. For instance, when you're in too steep and you want to sideslip down the mountain a bit, it's very important that you feel the snow with your feet, to make sure your footing is solid and balanced. When you're skiing in deep powder, you have to feel that your feet and knees are as close together as possible. Don't look at the ski tips—*feel* them. Some inner-skiing instructors suggest their students try skiing with their eyes closed, so as to experience the mountain moving underfoot. You'll also be able to feel your way through a parallel turn as a result of increasing body awareness. When you transfer your weight you should make that special effort to reach down with your mind and actually feel the bone of your foot pressing into the boot. It will do wonders for your control, your confidence . . . and, in the long *or* short run, your skiing.

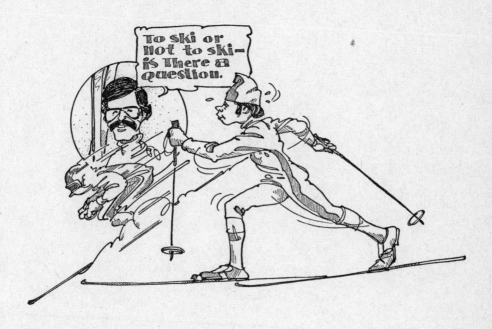

13. Racquet Sports

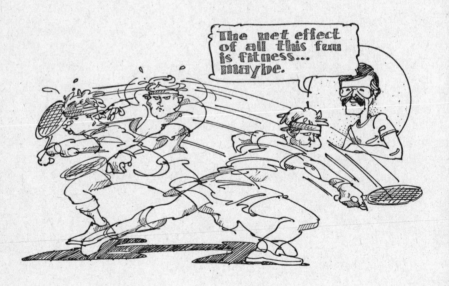

Dear Dr. Jock:

Can you help 34 women? There are a whole bunch of us in a tennis league and several of us are having a terrible time with tennis elbow. Here is what the group wants to know: (1) How long does it last? (It seems like forever!) (2) Can we continue to play even if it's painful? (3) If we continue, can the damage become permanent? (4) What kind of treatment will ease the pain? (5) Will it ever, ever, ever go away?

The Titusville 34, Titusville, Florida

Dear Dr. Jock:

I'm 54, 6'1", normal weight, and I've been playing tennis pretty regularly about twenty years. All of a sudden now, when I serve or lift my arm to hit an overhead return, I feel a sharp pain in my shoulder, right on the shoulder blade. It only hurts when I play but some days the pain is unbearable. The thought of giving up tennis is horrendous but I don't know what to do. What could be my problem?

D.M., Kansas City, Kansas

Dear Dr. Jock:

I'm not going to tell you how much I weigh but it's too much, believe me. I want to get started on an exercise program and really get myself in shape and I heard that racquetball burns up more calories than tennis and is better for you, too. Is this true? Is it dangerous? (I am 78.)

S.F., Chicago, Illinois

A lot of nerve we have, callously lumping all the racquet sports together as though tennis, racquetball, squash, badminton and that racquet game without a racquet, handball, were all just alike. They're not of course. They each go at their own pace, with their own rules, rewards and requirements. But they have a few important things in common, some shared ingredients that help distinguish them from any of the other popular sports.

The racquet sports require speed, agility and endurance. And intelligence. They're Thinking Games, all of them, with bigger stakes psychologically, because at the end there is a winner and a loser. That ain't necessarily so in swimming, or running, or riding a bike.

The racquet sports are competitive games that require you to think about offense as well as defense, sports that require you to be keenly aware of your opponent's moves and to plan your own several steps in advance. You can have a good time without doing either but your game will suffer. Your body may too.

In running and swimming, your mind can play around more, and while your body is moving at its own rhythmical pace, you are free to quietly dwell on tomorrow's loan presentation or let your mind wander to the beach at Maui. That's called dissociation and it's standard operating procedure in some sports.

But that kind of thinking can destroy your tennis and wreck your racquetball because racquet sports are games of strategy and concentration. To play your best, to be as good as you want to be, all the physical and mental energy you can muster must be present and accounted for. You have to know all the moves, sure, but you have to be able to use the moves when you need them, and you have to know when you need them. When you get good enough, you can play by instinct and that's part of the special draw of tennis, of racquetball, of squash, etc.—they can be such a total involvement, so all-consuming. But this means you have to concentrate. You have to be aware. You have to tune the rest of the world out. "When I play tennis, I'm a different person," one friend puts it. "I give myself totally to the game. I think of nothing else. I used to think sometimes about how much money tennis was costing me in day care, but it was ruining my game. Now I just think about the tennis, and when I'm really playing well, I don't even think about that." That's why she's so good, and perhaps why an hour of fast tennis or racquetball can be so refreshing, so ultimately relaxing.

The racquet sports can be very unrelaxing, however, even acutely anxiety producing, if you don't keep winning in perspective. Sure, you should play to win, and if you're a competition player, winning may be the only payoff you'll be happy with. But the biggest victory as you grow older is to be able to play the game well, play it regularly and have a good time at it. If you can do that, you'll keep going to a ripe old age, and if you keep going and stay active, you can't lose.

Which brings us to another point in all the racquet sports' favor: they are fun. You may take up swimming because, Lord knows, it's good for you, and you may get into running because it's the thing to do, but if tennis or racquetball or squash or handball become a habit, it's probably because you're having a heckuva good time. And that's what you should be looking for. To play. To have fun. To be a child again, without cares, without responsibilities, with a wonderful game to play.

The racquet sports are good for that, but what are they doing to your fitness? The answer depends on you: how much, how hard do you play? If you dabble in a slow, sociable game of doubles every Tuesday night and supplement occasionally with an hour of singles Sunday morning with your wife, then your tennis game isn't going to get you in condition. In fact, you'll have to make a special effort to get into condition for it or, as you get older, you'll surely wind up with an overuse problem. Indeed, more than 50 percent of tennis players over 35 are expected to develop tennis elbow because they haven't equipped their bodies for the stress of tennis. If your case is bad enough, it may make you give up the game altogether. So if you're reading this and you're in the ranks of the occasional player, the lackadaisical tennis-lover, the "What, me worry?" player who never got beyond a lob-and-shuffle game, you'd better look to other sports to get you into shape.

But if you take your fun seriously, and play regularly, a racquet sport can help take you to a greatly improved level of fitness. If you tend to play singles, and if you play at a level that keeps the ball in play long enough to keep your feet moving and your heart racing, and if you play at least 3 times a week (or mix it up with other good conditioning sports, like cycling, swimming, running), then the net effect of all that activity can be quite positive in terms of cardiovascular fitness and overall body tone.

RACQUETBALL VS. TENNIS

One reason why racquetball has caught on across the country—especially with women—is that it offers the average recreational player a much faster workout than is likely in the average recreational game of tennis. Tennis may be more elegant, requiring more finesse and subtlety, but racquetball can't be beat when it comes to working up a sweat. You can learn the basics in a relatively short time and then an hour of the game can have you feeling absolutely wiped out. In tennis, unless you are a fairly good player with an equally strong opponent, you may spend a lot of time chasing balls, getting ready, waiting, walking around and staring into space. Racquetball is played in so confined a space that you're continually in motion. David prefers tennis; Marilynn swears by racquetball. Your preference is your business, and our business is helping you play it better and enjoy it more.

BETTER CONDITIONING, BETTER TENNIS

Since tennis is the more popular game (we've seen estimates that range from 11 million to 35 million players, with one expert predicting that there would be 80 million of them in the U. S. by the 1980s), we'll concentrate on it. But what we have to say about physical conditioning, injury prevention and mental readiness applies equally to all the other racquet sports.

Technique, skill and strategy are the cornerstones of anybody's game. If you bring a strong, flexible, well-conditioned body to your game, you'll fare much better than the tennis player who does nothing else to build strength or endurance. Members of the Davis Cup team run, a lot of pros lift weights and jump rope, and Stan Smith is very keen on 50-to-100-yard sprinting. Chapter 3 tells you what you need to know about setting up a fitness program for yourself.

TENNIS ELBOW

You'll know it when you get it. Lightning bolts of pain shoot down your arm when you lift a book, turn a doorknob, cut your meat or brush your teeth. Sometimes the pain when you play tennis gets so fierce you have to quit altogether. Tennis elbow, a form of tendinitis, is one of the most common injuries among tennis players and certainly the most talked about. Cures, remedies and suggested treatments range from copper bracelets to acupuncture; proposals involving wooden rackets and elaborate counterbraces are continually being served up; and still the malady lingers on.

What is tennis elbow, anyway? It's an inflammation of the tendon and of the muscles in the forearm that extend the fingers and wrist. The bony prominence you can feel on the outside of the elbow, known to anatomists as the lateral epicondyle of the humerus, is where all the extensor muscles originate and where the tendon attaches. Another kind of tennis elbow involves pain at the medial epicondyle, on the inside of the elbow. Called the pro's tennis elbow—it's not often seen in recreational players—it affects the muscles that flex the wrist and the fingers.

You can get tennis elbow from other things besides tennis. Politicians may get it by shaking too many hands, and so can gamblers who shoot craps too vigorously. So can woodchoppers, football players, golfers and luggage handlers. David got the flexor version one year when he went cross-country skiing, from using his poles wrong, and his wife June did in her elbow by carrying heavy water buckets to her horses.

No matter how the problem originates, the cause is the same: too much stress, too little strength. Like every sort of tendinitis, it is an overuse syndrome, a build-up of microscopic tears until one day the system breaks down. If you get it, it's because your arm isn't strong enough, or flexible enough, to handle the stress and pressure of the workout you gave it. It could be, also, that you're hitting your backhand all wrong. If so, you've got lots of company.

If you're used to hitting with your girlfriend Sandy and then you go away for two weeks of much harder play with your husband, you are putting more stress on your forearm than it is ready for, and you could wind up with a ravaging case of tennis elbow. Anyone with a weak, flabby or undeveloped forearm is susceptible and so is the person who has started to smack the ball hard without warming up first. The looser, more lubricated your arm is before you play, the better able it is to adjust to stress without causing muscle or tendon tears. Age is another factor since, as we get older, our muscles naturally get tighter. Tennis elbow is much more common in the 35-and-older group, and if you fit in there, you'd better take charge and stay loose before it's too late.

It's never too late to correct your sloppy backhand punch, a common mistake in tennis that contributes to many cases of tennis elbow. Tennis is not an easy, or even an inexpensive sport to learn, but if you don't learn to hit a proper backhand, more than your game will suffer. Strong, able players know that you're not supposed to push or poke at the ball with your elbow when you're hitting a backhand. Your elbow should be tucked in and pointing toward the ground, not the net. Your source of power is your upper arm and your shoulder, not your forearm and wrist. The ideal backhand (and you shouldn't count on learning this from a book—you need a pro or learned friend to help you experience what we're talking about) is done with your front shoulder down and rotated and your elbow down too, and as you swing through the ball, you shift your weight from the back foot to the front foot. That's where a major portion of the real power comes from. Poor players try and muscle the shot over. Or they try and make a return shot with the ball too far in front of their body, or too far behind. In both cases the dynamics of hitting the ball puts too much stress on your tender tendon attachments. You unconsciously overload the circuits, overuse the system, and the resulting breakdown is tennis elbow.

LEG INJURIES

Tears in the calf muscle, hamstring pulls and injuries to the Achilles tendon are other major injuries for tennis players to watch out for. Racquet sports involve a lot of quick starts and desperate lunges, and if your muscles aren't loose and flexible enough, you can do real harm to your calf muscle. If that happens, put ice on the injured spot as soon as you can, to reduce the bleeding and swelling. Wrapping it with an elastic bandage and keeping it elevated will help hold down swelling too. A shoe with an elevated heel may make it easier to walk. A pull, a tear, a violent rip are problems for your doctor to consider—you'll need a specific diagnosis. If he confirms your worst suspicions, expect to be off the court for at least six weeks and don't go back until you have regained full flexibility and strength in the injured muscle. How do you know when that is? When it is equal in strength, in flexibility, in range of pain-free motion to its counterpart on the other side.

If the diagnosis is a torn Achilles tendon, you have a major injury and one that will probably leave you with some permanent disability. The Achilles tendon is one of the strongest in the body. It can stand a lot of force and won't tear unless it is, for some reason, abnormal. In operating on Achilles tendons that have been torn, David has always found that the tendon is degenerated in some way. Nobody knows what causes the degeneration; but once it happens, you're much more vulnerable to injury. Most people who tear an Achilles tendon have never noticed any symptoms before it happens. If yours is torn, you'll know right away that you're in trouble. You may be able to walk but you won't be able to stand on tiptoes. The heel will swell up fast, and if you put your finger on it at the back you may feel an actual dent where the tendon once was. The injury requires a cast or surgery; most sports-medicine experts advise surgery since it is likelier to give you more playing strength for the future. But some surgeons believe they get just as good a result with a cast. If that is the choice, you'll be in a cast for at least six weeks, more likely three months. And you'll have to work hard in a formal program of physical therapy afterward to recover enough motion and strength to get back to your regular game. You can do it, though.

SHOULDER PROBLEMS

There is one more nemesis for tennis players, especially older ones. With age, the power muscles in the shoulder get shorter, thicker and more inflexible unless there is a special effort to keep them stretched and strong.

Just as with tennis elbow, shoulder problems are overuse problems. When you serve hard, or lift your shoulder high to prepare for an overhand smash return, it is easy to cause small tears in the tendons or to pinch them between the head of the humerus and the acromion process, the bony prominence on top of your shoulder. In that case, you end up with a tendinitis, and that hurts.

Also, to make things more complicated, a bursa that lies just over the tendons at the top of the shoulder can also get inflamed. Sometimes it's hard to differentiate between a bursitis and a tendinitis, but the best treatment for either one is ice and aspirin. If the pain gets worse, you'd better see your doctor.

PREVENTING INJURIES

We don't have a cure for tennis elbow. There are things you can do to prevent it, however. The same goes for injuries to the leg and shoulder.

WARM UP BEFORE YOU PLAY

This is the key to preventing all overuse injuries, and it is absolutely essential in tennis. (See our list of recommended warm-ups in Chapter 7.) If you've only got an hour's court time, do 10 minutes of stretching before you get out there. Do it slowly and gently; be aware of any spots where you have special tension. Stretch out the calves, the hamstrings, the shoulders—all the body parts you'll be using. The wall lean is a good stretch for the calf, and doing toe raises with weights (described in Chapter 8) will stretch as well as strengthen your calf muscles. Jumping rope for 10 minutes or so is a good way to get the juices flowing, too. You should do flexibility exercises every day, whether you play tennis or not, but to play without stretching first is lunacy. Then, when you get onto the court, don't begin at maximum strength. Ease into your best game.

STRENGTHEN THE FOREARM MUSCLES

Every other day, take 10 minutes to work on strengthening the flexors and extensors. If your forearm is strong and ready for action, the chances of developing tennis elbow are greatly reduced. You'll find some special strengthening exercises at the end of this chapter.

TAKE LESSONS

Learn the proper strokes and practice them until they become second nature. Then you can concentrate on other things, such as strategy and placement. (Your lousy backhand may be good enough to pop the ball over the net most times, but it can also be a major cause of tennis elbow.)

CHOOSE YOUR RACQUET CAREFULLY

A grip that is too small will twist in your hand, and one that is too large will be tough to control, and tiring to your hand and forearm muscles. Let the pro at your shop guide you, but one general hint is that the distance from the tip of your middle finger to the middle crease of your palm is about the right circumference for your racquet handle. You should also be able to insert your index finger between the tip of your middle finger and the base of your thumb when you hold the racquet. If you can't do that, it's probably the wrong size.

The debate over metal vs. wooden racquets won't be settled here, but keep in mind that the more flexible your racquet is, the more it can absorb vibrations and the shock of play. A very rigid racquet may aggravate the situation, as will hitting with one that is so heavy in the head that you have trouble meeting the ball out in front of you. A lighter racquet may be a better choice for beginners. No racquet will, all by itself, keep you from getting tennis elbow. It's an accumulation of factors, complicated by your *own* benign neglect of the basics.

MAKE SURE YOUR RACQUET IS STRUNG TO THE RIGHT TENSION

Bjorn Borg may have his strung to 70 pounds, but the odds are your arm can't take that kind of pressure. If it's strung too tight, more force is transmitted to the arm, and the greater the risk of tennis elbow becomes. For most people, from 52 to 56 pounds of tension is about right.

COPING WITH PAIN

Once you get tennis elbow, or any other tendinitis, all you can really do is wait for it to heal itself. That could take months; it could take a year or more. The disease is self-limiting, which means that it will eventually go away by itself. Meanwhile, it won't make much difference if you go on playing (or shaking hands, or chopping wood, or shooting craps), so long as the pain is bearable. When it ceases to be, that is usually the time to go to a doctor—not to speed up the healing time (your doctor can't do that), but to get a pain-killer or anti-inflammatory medication. All the standard treatments for tendinitis are geared to relieving or disguising the pain.

If you go on playing, it may help to use a heating pad, or to run hot water from the tap over the sore part beforehand. Some people like to keep a sore elbow extra warm by having it covered while they play. It may help to wear a snug elastic band that you can buy in a sports shop. Many players wear this device too high, or else too low, or too tight. It should hug the arm, just below the elbow and tendon attachment. It eases the injured and vulnerable spot by diffusing some of the force you expend over a larger area, taking the pressure and tension off the muscle attachment. The less pressure, the less pain. At least, that's the theory.

If you go back to playing with shoulder tendinitis, and don't have a clear awareness of what caused the problem in the first place, you're likely to repeat the injury. To avoid that, spend a few minutes every day doing exercises to increase shoulder flexibility, in addition to warming up faithfully every time you play. If the shoulder continues to bother you, slow down your game. Play smart instead of tough. Try to avoid using your arm overhead, a motion that may pinch the already swollen tendons. Ease up on your serve and place it better.

After you play, you can cut down inflammation and pain by putting an ice pack on the elbow or shoulder 3 or 4 times a day, 15 or 20 minutes at a time. Aspirin may also help; some players take it *before* they play, so they won't feel the pain as much during the game. Then there are the nondrug ways of dealing with pain—relaxation, deep breathing and visualization. You'll have to experiment and find what works for you.

If the pain becomes too intense, you may decide to see a doctor who has an interest in sports medicine and discuss the possibility of a shot of cortisone. But be aware of the drawbacks (more about this in Chapter 16). David's policy is to limit his patients to two or three injections a year. If you decide on a shot of cortisone, you shouldn't go back to tennis until after about ten days of nonplaying, body-healing time, no matter how dramatic the relief.

PROTECT YOUR EYES

In racquetball, in squash, in all the racquet sports, you've got to keep your eye on the ball. And that brings us to the issue of eye injuries and eye protectors. A serious eye injury is a real possibility in the fast racquet sports, and you ought to wear protective lenses of some sort, especially if you're wearing contact lenses when you play. Tennis and badminton players can probably get by with ordinary street spectacles that have nonbreakable lenses, but racquetball and squash players need more protection than that. There are several good devices on the market for you to choose from: try a few and see which one feels most comfortable and least obtrusive.

Too often the injury occurs *after* the point is over and your guard is down, when the other player has a tantrum and takes one last angry crack at the ball—and you end up with seven stitches in your eye. One way to avoid such problems is to play defensively. Be aware of the ball but don't set yourself up as an easy target. Use your peripheral vision, or your racquet face, to protect yourself. If you still feel queasy about your evasive tactics, get advice from a pro.

Finally, learn to control your own temper when you're on the court so you don't become the cause of someone else's eye injury. Hurling your racquet skyward, or kicking the racquetball, is infantile. It blows your concentration and makes you a dangerous player besides.

FINE-TUNING YOUR GAME

Concentration is everything in racquet games. You may have a kill shot from the back court that is deadly, an absolutely devastating net game or a return of serve that can leave your opponent in tears, but unless you've learned to concentrate on the court, you're not getting all you can out of your game. Concentration can turn a poor player into a good one, and make a good one better.

Concentration on the court means that all your attention is directed toward maximizing your strengths, toward keeping the ball in play long enough for you to win the point or for your opponent to lose it.

If you're up against a fast player, you've got to concentrate on slowing him down. Against one who is hitting easy, holding back for a strong finish, concentrate on conserving your own energy too. In doubles, you need to concentrate on communicating with your partner, anticipating needs, staying in synch, on the same wavelength.

Concentration, like any other discipline, takes practice and willpower. You should start the focusing process in your warm-ups before the game begins. Direct your thoughts and feelings to your calves, your knees, your shoulders and your back. Are they loose? Are you ready for action? Are there any tension spots you've missed? During the game, if you feel your concentration dissipating, refocus by taking a few deep breaths; tie your shoelaces, or stare at the tennis ball, or call out "bounce-hit" to yourself every time the ball bounces and you go after it.

Don't, however, confuse saying "bounce-hit" or "racquet back" with a lot of futile chatter about how you're *not* getting your racquet back, or *not* watching the ball, or *not* hitting to your opponent's backhand. Don't pollute the still waters with incriminating remarks. Don't nag or harp or criticize—you'll only get in your own way. Play ball. Your body already knows what to do. Your job is not getting in its way. And most of all, your job is to enjoy.

You will enjoy the game 100 percent more if you can learn one of the hardest lessons of all, to keep your eye on the ball—or, as our tennis-teaching friend, David Hacker says, keep your eye on where the ball *has been*. In fast play, the ball is hitting and bouncing off your racquet much too fast for you actually to see the action. A good player keeps his or her eye on where the ball has been, finishes the stroke and then follows the flight of the ball across the court. If you snap your head back too fast, not only will you miss what you couldn't see to begin with, but you'll compromise your stroke.

One good exercise for improving hand-eye coordination is to try bouncing a tennis ball against the ground, using the edge of your racquet instead of the flat. Another is the Shadow Drill, a concentration increaser, highly recommended by Carol Kleiman in her book, *You Can Teach Your Child Tennis*. If, when you're playing, you blow a return or miss the ball altogether, instead of tossing your racquet away or smacking down your fist, run through the stroke you just missed, repeating it physically and visualizing it mentally. That will get you right back into the game.

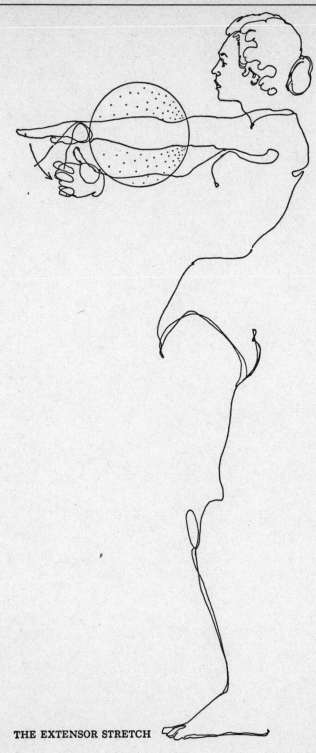

THE EXTENSOR STRETCH

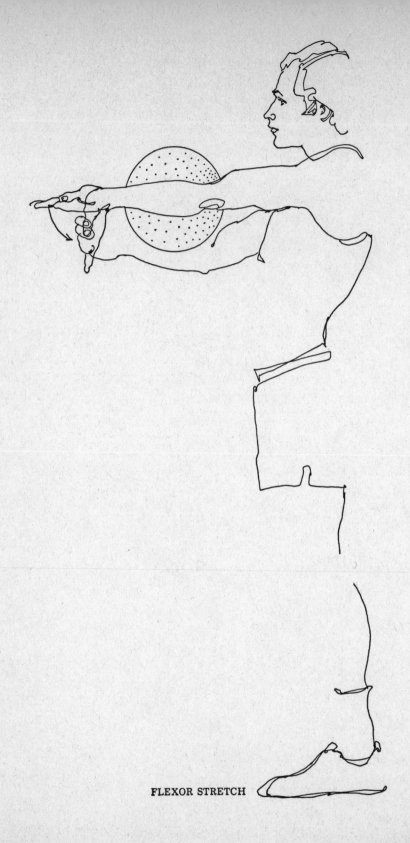

FLEXOR STRETCH

EXERCISES TO PREVENT TENNIS ELBOW

THE EXTENSOR STRETCH

Hold your arm out, palm down, elbow straight, fingers extended. Bend your wrist down as far as you can, using your other hand to push it farther. Feel the stretch, and hold it for 5 seconds. Repeat 5 times.

FLEXOR STRETCH

This is the same as the Extensor Stretch except that you do it with your palm up. With your elbow straight, bend your wrist *down* as far as you can, and use your other hand to push down farther. Keep your fingers pointing down, straight to the floor. Feel the stretch and hold for 5 seconds. Repeat 5 times.

FOREARM STRENGTHENER

Squeezing a ball or one of those hand-grip devices is a fine way to strengthen the flexor muscles, but it won't do much for the extensors—and that's where most people have problems. Fingertip push-ups will help with both, but not everyone can do them. If you can, go right ahead.

AN ISOMETRIC

Hold your arm out straight with your fingers extended, and hold them there as hard as you can while you use your other hand to try to bend your fingers and wrist. Or put your arm under an immovable object, such as a heavy table, to get the same kind of pressure and resistance. Once you get in position, at maximum resistance, hold it for at least 5 seconds and repeat 5 times. Do this with your wrist and hand at several different angles.

USE YOUR RACQUET TO BUILD STRENGTH

You can use your racquet with the press, or with a weighted cover, to build strength in your forearm. Hold the racquet by the end of the handle, arm out straight and palm down. Lift the racquet head up as high as you can by bending your wrist back. Repeat slowly, as often as you can. Try to work up, gradually, to 25 times.

WEIGHTS

A 5-pound dumbbell is a good investment. Sit with your hand over the edge of a table or chair arm. Holding the weight with your palm down will allow you to work on your extensor muscles; palm up works the flexors. Move your wrist up and down as far as you can. Do as many repetitions as possible.

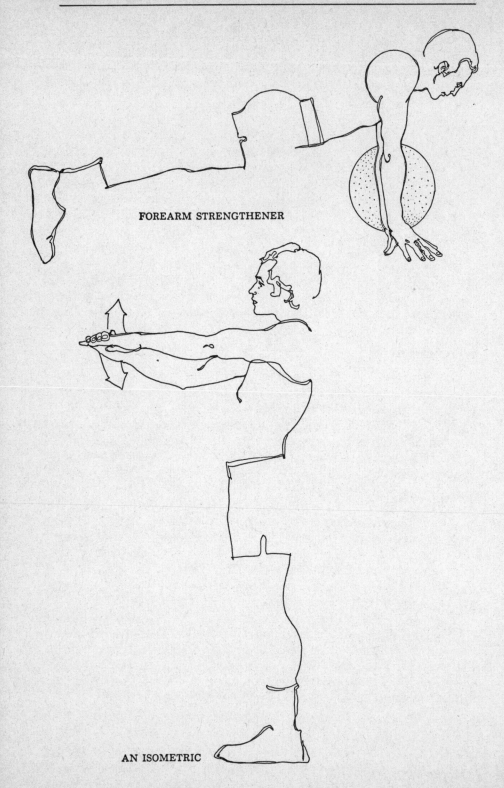

FOREARM STRENGTHENER

AN ISOMETRIC

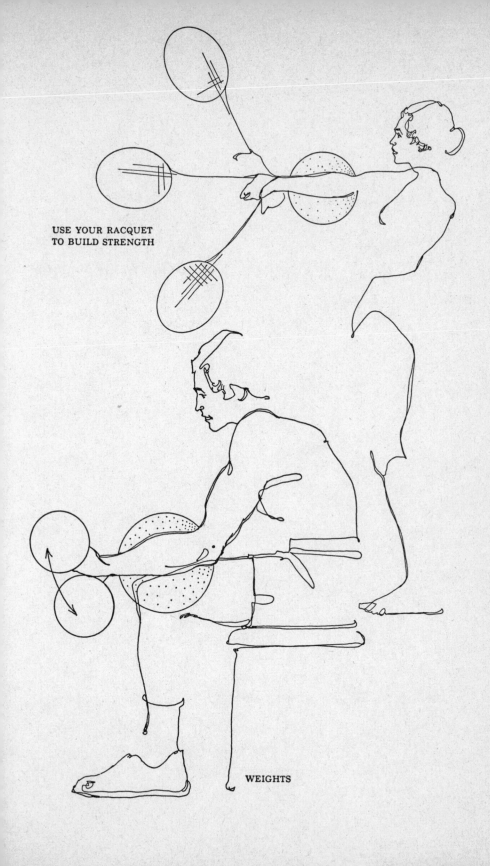

USE YOUR RACQUET
TO BUILD STRENGTH

WEIGHTS

14. Golf

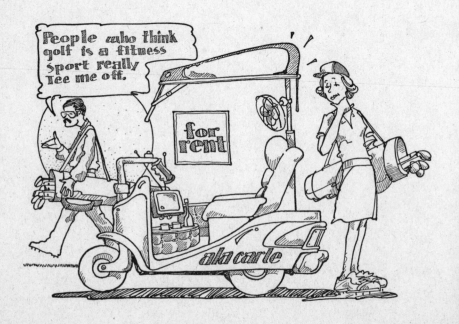

Dear Dr. Jock:

I've been having a lot of trouble with my back lately, and I'm wondering if I should continue to play golf. Does golf aggravate the condition? Is there anything that would make it better? I sure hate to give up my game (I've been in the same foursome twenty-seven years), but my back is getting so bad I don't know what to do.

K.L., Detroit, Michigan

Dear Dr. Jock:

I played golf in college, then I quit the game for about ten years and now I'm getting back into it. But I'm running into a real problem: frequently, when I hit the ball, I feel a very sharp pain on the outside of my left elbow. It's getting so bad I'm beginning to dread going out. Do you have any idea what I might be doing wrong?

W.R., Chicago, Illinois

Dear Dr. Jock:

Can you settle an argument, please? My friend is an avid 3-times-a-week golfer and he says that's just as good a way to stay in condition as my running program (3 miles, 3 times a week). I think he's wrong and we bet a 6-pack, so please let us know who's right as soon as possible. Thanks.

JM., Los Angeles, California

Golf is an enormously popular game in this country. It requires balance, coordination, power, patience and an uncanny ability to keep that eye on the ball. If you lose your focus, or think too much, or try too hard, you're in trouble. And keeping out of trouble, away from traps, bunkers, rough, deep woods, hooks, slices, flubs, mishits and all the other errors and uncertainties that plague the average golfer, is the secret of a successful game.

However, no matter how many millions play it and no matter how hard they defend its subtle mysteries, golf is not a fitness sport. In short, if you play it and only it, and don't do any other exercise or play any other sport, you will not condition your cardiovascular system. Golf doesn't fit the three requirements of duration, intensity and endurance. It may challenge your psyche and exhaust your energy, but it can't really do much to tone up sagging muscles or help you lose weight. That's the bad news.

The good news is that golf is a fascinating, challenging game. It can involve some 4 to 5 miles of walking—if you resist the *a la carte* temptations—and it can offer you a few, quiet hours to get away, relax and contemplate the joys and frustrations of trying to batter, bully and coax a little white ball into a tiny round hole. During the course of a game, you can probably burn up 400 to 500 calories, but if you're not careful, you'll easily eat up that much and possibly more if you celebrate the 19th hole with too many beers and peanuts.

If you're scrounging for reasons to justify the time you spend at golf, you'll be happy to hear that a kinesiologist at the University of Waterloo in Canada has testified that golf "has a very important role in maintaining the level of the oxidative enzymes in the slow twitch muscles especially."

And perhaps, if you are already in tip-top shape when you play golf, it may help you maintain the condition of the upper-body muscles. But don't look to golf as a game to get you into shape, not unless you play it 4 or 5 times a week and combine it with a serious weight-training, weight-loss regimen. Most people who play golf, though, don't do that. They just play golf. And they're lucky if they can get out once a week. And *if* they get out once a week, they probably won't walk the course and carry their bag. They'll probably pull a golf cart or, even more conducive to sloth, ride an electric cart.

If you play and you're looking for ways to get a little more exercise out of your game, you should start by swearing off the electric golf cart. If the club you play at insists on one, get a friend, or obliging family member to drive behind you as you walk the course—doctor's orders. If you're not used to so much walking, work up to it gradually. Walk a hole, ride a hole; do whatever you have to do to gradually accustom your body to walking the full 9 or 18 holes. If you work up to carrying your bag, too, all the better. And if you ever get to the point where you can hit the ball, change to running shoes, pick up your bag and carry it from shot to shot, hole to hole, that's when you'll be using golf to boost your fitness level too.

LET GOLF CHALLENGE YOU, NOT DEFEAT YOU

In the meantime, you should watch what golf does to your anxiety level. It's not a high-risk sport in terms of injuries, and most of the ones that golfers do suffer are related to stress and anxiety brought on by the game. Golfers can be an excitable, competitive lot. The ones who appear loose and relaxed, the way Gene Littler does, are in the minority. The tension in their minds carries over into their muscles—and tense muscles are more easily sprained, strained and pulled. Anxious golfers inevitably compromise their game. So the first thing you should do to better your game and cut down the risk of injury is to learn how to handle stress. Don't let your anxieties about winning, about losing, about the long waits between holes, about the bunkers and water holes that are lurking all around the course, ready to swallow up your best drive of the day, get the best of you. Chapter 5, on mental conditioning, will help you understand why you need to practice relaxation before, during, even after you play. It's okay to compare yourself to other players and it's nice to know that other people admire your ability. But if you let your ego take over your game, you're going to get hurt. If you compete with yourself and keep your sense of humor, you can't come up a loser.

One sure way to cut down on golfer's anxiety is to take the time and make the effort to learn the basics of the game. Sand traps are less stress-inducing if you know how to blast your way out. The whole game becomes more fun once you're confident that you know the proper swing. It's possible to learn, difficult to perfect, and there are an infinite number of subtle variations. Taking golf lessons is just like taking a few minutes to calm yourself down before you play—it's a precaution.

Everyone who takes up golf learns approximately the same sort of swing. It's no real mystery, it's all in the books and you can see it repeated dozens of times every weekend—sometimes even broken down into slow motion—on your home TV screen. It seems so simple, so smooth, so possible. All you have to do is keep your head down, your left hand firm, swing under and out, and finish high, with your belly-button headed for the flag. And, oh yes, keep your eye on the ball. That's what you know—but that isn't what you should think about just before you hit. Some experts say you're better off *not* to think. Your body already knows how to swing the club. Trust your body; trust yourself. And above all, steer your mind clear of its natural tendency to nag ("head down, hand firm, swing under, finish high," and so on), and focus instead on something more positive, more productive. Turn your mind's eye toward a mental movie-of-your-own-creation, and watch your golf ball fly down the course, headed for the hole, as high and straight and as far as you want to carry it. It's only a fantasy and it only takes a few seconds' thought, so why not try it the next time you tee off? Or perhaps next time you're looking for a little, looping 9-iron from the edge of the bunker? If you're having a hard time conjuring up an image of yourself sending the ball clear down the fairway, maybe you can get a picture of Alan Shepard's famous 6-iron on the moon, and how that ball just sailed and sailed and sailed.

Visualization of this kind may not improve your shots right away, but if you learn to do it right, it will undoubtedly relax you. And if your mind and muscles are at ease before you stroke the ball, you will unquestionably cut down on the aches and pains.

Here's another visualization that might be helpful:

> Imagine a golf ball. Make the image of it as vivid as you can. When anything intrudes upon the image, let it pass. If the golf ball disappears, imagine it again. If it wavers, make it steady. Doing this, you can practice keeping your eye on the ball. You can practice it in your room on a rainy day. If you cannot keep something out of your mind, some hive out of your soul-skin, when you are practicing this inner sight, get to know the intrusion. What does it show you about yourself and your situation in the world? Exploring the invader can be helpful to your game.

The passage is from a fascinating book by the sports yoga pioneer Michael Murphy, called *Golf in the Kingdom*. It's an example of what we mean when we talk about conjuring up a mental picture that will help you focus all your awareness and energy on the game at hand. You can try it any time, or better, you can try one of your own. According to the golf columnist and psychiatrist, Dr. John Morley,

> What most people don't realize is that we have more control over nervousness and tension than we think we do. The key to getting rid of anxiety is to use one's imagination. The golfer should think of his body as a receptacle filled with psychic fluid representing the anxiety. He should let this fluid drain out of his system beginning at the top of his head and moving right down through the tip of the toes. This only takes about fifteen seconds; the golfer needn't worry. This technique has been used in hypnotic procedures for years and it can reduce tension much faster than any tranquilizer. The more one practices this, the more effective he becomes in getting rid of tension and anxiety.

GOLF ELBOW

Tennis players aren't the only ones. Virtually the same ailment as tennis elbow also happens to golfers. And it hurts. Most often it is caused by an improper swing. You take your swing and before it reaches the ball (if, in fact, it ever does reach the ball) the clubhead slams into the ground, and your lead, or pulling arm, is clobbered. The extensor muscles of the wrist and hand are tightly wrapped around the club as it swings one way—and then suddenly they are jolted back and forced the other way. Small tears in the tendon attachment at the elbow can be the result. After repeated mishits and the resulting stresses, scar tissue forms in the tendon. This can really hurt, like a dagger sticking into your elbow every time you connect with the ball. Since golf elbow affects the nondominant arm—if you're a right-handed golfer you'll feel it in your left elbow, and vice versa—it usually doesn't cause as much trouble or inconvenience as tennis elbow does to tennis players. An ice pack on your elbow for 15 or 20 minutes after you play will reduce swelling and thus ease the pain. If you can, warm up your elbow with a heating pad or warm water before going out on the course. It's not dangerous to go on playing, so long as the pain isn't so bad that it takes away all the fun. To prevent this kind of golf elbow, the main thing is learning to hit the ball properly. The arm-strengthening exercises at the end of Chapter 13, "Racquet Sports," will also help.

Another kind of golfer's elbow happens to the inside of the elbow, and involves the tendons of the flexor muscles of the wrist and hand. Good golfers who regularly take too big a divot when they hit their iron shots may come up with this ailment. When too much strain is placed on the tendon, it may rebel—especially if it's weak and relatively inflexible. Again, ice is the best treatment; better technique and stronger muscles, the best prevention.

SHOULDER TENDINITIS

Most of us don't have great flexibility in the shoulders to begin with, since so few tasks require us to lift our arms over our head and stretch and twist our shoulders through a full range of motion. And—as we keep telling you—the older we get, the less flexible we are. The golf swing, then, can really take its toll on your shoulders if you're not careful. If your muscles and tendons are tight and unused to working around the back and over the head, swinging your golf club can cause microscopic tears. You may not feel each one of these, but thick scar tissue can form as they heal—and when that tears, you're in big trouble. Thickened scar tissue is also liable to being pinched between the head of the humerus (the upper arm bone) and the acromion process (the bony prominence on the top of the shoulder).

Shoulder tendinitis may be a constant aching pain or a sharp stabbing pain when you use the arm. In either case, the treatment is the same: ice to reduce the swelling, aspirin to relieve the pain and help ease the inflammation. Eventually, as the body heals, the pain will go away—though not as quickly as it arrived. If, in the meantime, the pain becomes really bad, you'll want to see a doctor. This is one place where a shot of hydrocortisone often gives dramatic relief.

To prevent the trouble in the first place, keep your shoulders flexible all during the year. As you stand waiting for an elevator or a bus, or for the water to boil, stretch your shoulder muscles through the full range of motion. Keep a golf club handy in your office, your car or your kitchen, and at least once a day grab it with both hands and loosen the tension in the shoulder muscles by holding it over and behind your head. This exercise should be part of the stretching warm-up before you play. Strengthening exercises in themselves aren't particularly helpful with this problem.

HAND AND WRIST PROBLEMS

Remember the time you were on the par-3, 220-yard hole, and all you could think of was how hard you'd like to wallop that ball? You wound up like a coiled spring and let loose with a swing that smashed your clubhead into the ground so hard that your wrists felt as though they'd been jammed into a concrete wall. Things like that can take the fun away from golf. Most often, hand and wrist injuries are the result of mishitting the ball. You may sprain the wrist itself, or perhaps the fragile metacarpal bones of the ring and little fingers. Since a sprain is an injury and not an overuse syndrome, the best treatment is resting the hand until it heals. That could take three or four weeks. No matter how frustrating a wait that may be, if you go back too early, you can do more serious damage by reinjury.

BACK PAIN

Since the physical demands of golf aren't terribly great, it lends itself to out-of-shape, overweight, undisciplined participants. That's why we hear so frequently from golfers who complain that their backs hurt. The lateral shifts and twists of the lower back during the swing place an extra stress on the supporting muscles and ligaments. If those muscles aren't strong enough and enough stress is applied, the ligaments may not hold up, and the discs may even be damaged. Compound this with all the tension and anxiety golfers tend to feel anyway, and you've got a backache waiting to happen.

Since low back pain is so common—David calls it America's most widespread social disease—it's impossible to single out a cause. Frequently the problem is postural; if so, it may be correctable if you're willing to take responsibility, and do some work.

If you've been checked out by a doctor and there's no apparent abnormality in the back itself, start to work not on your back, but your stomach. Weak abdominal muscles are the reason for a lot of lower back pain. You'll understand why if you visualize your trunk as a cylinder, something like a soft-drink can. If one side caves in or balloons out (that's your stomach), extra stress is put on the metal of the other side (that's your back), and the cylinder may collapse.

The best way to prevent low back pain is to keep the whole cylinder strong—which often means working on weak, flabby stomach muscles.

To strengthen them, begin a lifelong habit of doing bent-leg sit-ups. Do them once a week, or as part of a pregame warm-up, but every single day. Make them part of your regular schedule—something you do every morning just after getting out of bed, or else as part of your going-to-bed routine. Start out slowly—it may be that 5 or 10 will be all you can handle comfortably at first. If you stick with the exercise, you'll add more and more, and by the time you get to 50 you may wonder whatever happened to those miserable backaches.

The best way to do the sit-ups is to lie on your back with the hips and knees flexed and the feet flat on the floor. Keep your arms at your side, or better yet, cross them over your chest. Begin the exercise from the sitting-up position; lean back as far as you can keep in control. Bent knee sit-ups are much better than doing sit-ups with your legs extended because they put less strain on your back. Bending the hips also relaxes the hip flexor muscles and gives the abdominal muscles more work to do. And the harder they work, the easier it'll be for you to continue your golf without having to worry about unnecessary low back pain.

Prevention of back pain is much more tolerable for most people than treatment. That's because the best treatment is rest, and if there's one thing an avid golfer likes less than a double-bogey on a par 3, it's having to stop golf altogether and rest. Lying down is the only way you can really rest your back, and even then you ought to make an effort specifically to work out the tension in your back muscles, since their tight, tense condition probably caused the backache in the first place.

Heat is sometimes soothing for a sore back but most people tend to overdo it. Back pain frequently can come from sprained joints and ligaments. As in all sprains, this is accompanied by swelling. Heat only increases swelling, so too much heat applied to a sore back may increase the pain. If you are going to use heat, limit it to 20 minutes at a time with the pad set on low and don't apply it more than 4 times a day. And *don't* sleep on a heating pad. That's one of those bits of folk medicine lore that has hung on in spite of all we know about treating sprains.

By the way, if the pain doesn't subside or you keep getting sciatica, pain down the back of the leg, abandon your self-care attempts and see your doctor. Numbness or weakness in the leg is a sign of more serious problems and requires expert advice. However, even your local medical expert is probably going to prescribe bed rest first thing, just to see if the body can be persuaded to heal itself.

HIP TENDINITIS

Tendinitis of the hip muscles bothers many golfers. It's actually a pain in the gluteus medius, the large muscle that runs from the pelvic rim to the top of the femur. This is the muscle that allows you to stand on just one leg. It is a strong one but the many lateral shifts and twists that golfing calls for may strain it, and repeated strains and tears may lead to tendinitis. The result will be pain in the upper and outer part of the thigh, which is aggravated by walking up or down stairs or hills. In time, like any tendinitis, it will heal naturally. Meanwhile, you can continue to play golf without harming yourself. The tricky part may be learning to overcome the pain so you can enjoy the game. If the pain gets intolerable and you feel disabled, you should see your doctor about a stronger, anti-inflammatory drug, or perhaps an injection of cortisone. Otherwise, self-treatment with ice and aspirin is made easier by knowing that in time this too shall pass.

WARM UP BEFORE YOU TEE OFF

To stretch out those hip muscles, hook your elbows around a club behind your back and twist your trunk each way as far as you can. This should help stretch your back muscles too. In another good stretch for the hips—it looks like an exaggerated hula motion—you stand with your weight on one leg and then thrust your hip as far as you can to the weighted leg side. Then shift your weight to the other leg—find your balance first, then thrust your hip in the opposite direction. You should feel a nice healthy pull in the hip area. The looser and more flexible all these muscles are before you go out to play, the less your risk of injury. A program of warm-ups especially designed for golfers is outlined in Chapter 7.

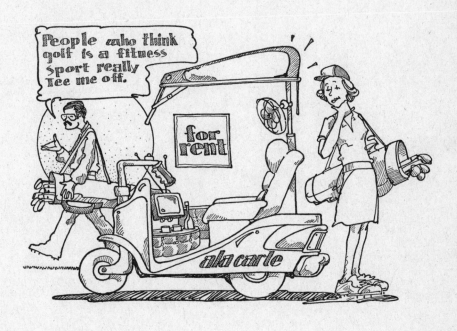

15. Bat and Ball

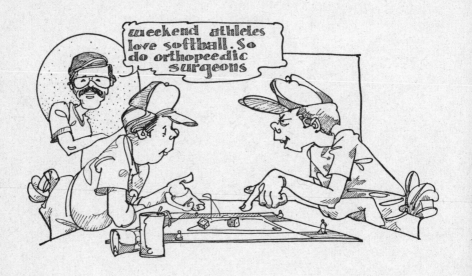

Games

Dear Dr. Jock:

My son is a pitcher in Little League. He likes it and I think it's done him a world of good. But lately, he's been coming home complaining that his pitching arm is sore. His coach says he'll be okay when he gets used to pitching. My son is afraid if he goes to a doctor the doctor will tell him to quit pitching, but I'm afraid of what might happen if he doesn't see a doctor. Is it normal to hurt? He is 12 and otherwise healthy. Thank you.

M.F., Akron, Ohio

Dear Dr. Jock:

I work at a company with a ladies' softball team. We compete in an industrial league. We don't know too much about the game but have a lot of fun playing, and afterwards we all go out and celebrate no matter which side won. What we're wondering is if there are some exercises we can do before we play to help us play better. (Our "coach" says the best thing we can do is get down on our knees and pray the other team doesn't show up!)

B.Y., Berwyn, Illinois

Dear Dr. Jock:

I play a lot of baseball (12", fast pitch) and last year and now again this year I had a real bad hamstring pull. Is this just old age (I'm 46) or what?

D.R., Wichita Falls, Texas

Is there an athlete alive who hasn't played baseball or softball? They're as all-American as apple pie and Sunday double-headers. The rules are pretty easy, the contact between players is minimal and the basic skills of hitting, throwing, catching are pretty much standard fare in every gym class in the country. Even in the darkest ages, when women were being held back from many other competitive sports, they could still play softball. In fact, everyone can play . . . or thinks they can. And that's part of the problem.

You'd think twice before strapping on a pair of skis and schussing down the Seiptoe Range in Sun Valley, but few of us bat an eye at having a few too many beers and joining the team at the company picnic.

It's not a game that requires you to be very fit to have fun, so while millions of people across America play it, many of them suffer costly injuries, aches and pains. We want you to keep on enjoying your baseball games, no matter what your level of skill or participation, and we want to tell you a few things that will help you enjoy them more. A little awareness and a few minutes of your time will make baseball more fun and even more important, as well as less risky. Softball may be just an occasional frolic, but a pulled hamstring is a pulled hamstring no matter how you get it. You can learn to avoid pulled hamstrings and a half-dozen of baseball's other most common injuries by taking a few precautions. Some are simple; some involve a lifelong commitment to good health and well-being. It's up to you to choose.

BASEBALL TEACHES TEAM PLAY

Baseball and softball are fun to play. That sense of play, that feeling of camaraderie that comes from playing on a team, is important in our lives. Baseball teaches us as much about cooperation as it does about coordination. The closer we get to nine or ten other players, the more we can learn about ourselves. Team sports teach you how to be a team player, and that seems to be excellent preparation for the game of Life. All that fanny-slapping and good-natured razzmatazzing carries over from the ball field to the board rooms, which is only one of many reasons why organized team sports are so important for women to learn. Baseball may help you pitch your ideas someday. It most certainly gives you experience in going to bat for yourself, and if sometimes you're caught stealing, well, at least the team can't say you didn't try. Everyone on Nixon's Watergate team could say they tried. So much for metaphors.

If playing baseball or softball isn't fun for you, something is seriously wrong. Maybe you're going in there all tense and nervous and ready to kill. If so, you're probably setting yourself up for major disappointments and at least minor injuries. A supercompetitive attitude is not the healthiest approach to take, especially not if you're a sometime recreational player. Play ball because you like it. It's fun.

Baseball is more a game than an exercise, and its benefits to the recreational player are mental and emotional rather than physical. Baseball and softball are not fitness sports. All by themselves, they won't do much to flatten your belly or improve lung capacity or trim flabby thighs. Baseball players tend to take a cavalier attitude toward such things and are not the fittest of athletes. Nevertheless, the better condition you're in before you play, the more you'll enjoy the game and the less likely you'll be to do something stupid and injure yourself.

In baseball, too many people think the pregame warm-up is the time players spend talking to TV sportscasters. You may not see the warm-ups before you hear the umpire call out "Play ball"—but they're happening. To make it happen for you, read Chapter 7.

WATCH YOUR LEGS

Speed, says Pete Rose, is the single greatest physical asset in baseball. Just being fast isn't enough, though. If you don't have flexibility too, you're going to suffer leg muscle pulls, one of the most common injuries in baseball. That sudden burst of speed when you're trying to stretch a strong single into a weak double can cause a tight hamstring to rip. Scrambling back to first base after a long leadoff, or lunging for a hard-hit grounder, can pull a groin muscle and leave you hobbling. A simple 10-minute warm-up that stretches the hamstrings, the groin and the calves will go a long way toward preventing these annoying injuries. For details on what to do if you're hurt on the field, be sure to read Chapter 4. You'll find there what you need to know about specific injuries and whether or not you can treat them at home or should see a doctor. Generally speaking, the treatment calls for complete healing and making sure normal flexibility is restored before returning to play. That may mean two days or two weeks or two months, depending on the severity of the injury.

DON'T BURN OUT YOUR ELBOW

Throwing a ball puts a great deal of stress on your arm. The throwing elbow of a professional pitcher eventually wears out. Like the fan belt in your car, the elbow is a mechanical part that can take only so much stress and strain. Most big league pitchers have abused it to the point of no return—many of them simply can't straighten out that arm anymore, as a result either of arthritis or contracture (a tightening of the capsule of the elbow joint, probably caused by overuse and chronic irritation).

The pros can rationalize a permanent injury—baseball is their bread and butter—but it's disturbing to see Little Leaguers in the doctor's office with a similar condition—dubbed Little League elbow—because somebody, either a parent or the coach or both, has allowed them to throw too hard for too long. Little League officials are attempting to deal with this serious problem by limiting the number of pitches a young person can throw. Parents should set limits also, especially on the amount of pushing they do when it comes to junior league sports. Behind many an injured youngster is a well-meaning mother or an overzealous dad, cheering him to victory and making him feel like a failure if he complains. Pushing a son or daughter that way can lead to an injury that may cause trouble for a lifetime. Remember that the next time your youngster comes home saying, "It hurts when I throw the ball." Kids are pretty flexible; it takes a lot for them to overuse a muscle or abuse a joint.

A Little League elbow can mean one of two things: either a problem (possibly tendinitis) on the inside of the elbow, where the flexor muscles of the hand and wrist attach to the humerus, or something more serious—for example, a piece of bone pulled away at the point of attachment, known as the medial epicondyle. Pain on the outside of the elbow may involve damage to the joint surface between the humerus and radius. In severe cases, when a fragment has broken away from the joint surface of the humerus, the elbow suddenly can't be straightened out. If any of these problems arise with your young pitcher, you should see an orthopedic surgeon immediately.

SHOULDERS NEED STRETCHING

Because (as we keep stressing) people tend to tighten up with age, and are especially unused to stretching out the shoulder muscles that are used in lifting the arms over the head to throw a ball, older ballplayers are likely to suffer from some shoulder pain. If you're bothered by this, be sure to warm up properly before you play (and do these same exercises every day, for best results). Stretch your shoulders through a full range of motion. And take it easy at the start, before you start to throw hard. If your shoulder begins to hurt during a game, it's possible to go on playing if you want to—but if the fun's all gone, and your team can do without you, you might as well head for the bench. Continue to stretch out those sore muscles if you can, and use an ice pack to cut down on swelling and pain. *Don't* run in from second base, aching and unhappy, and snuggle down with a heating pad. It might be helpful to warm up a muscle before you play; but after a game, it's the worst thing for an ailing, swollen muscle. Take aspirin for the pain. If the symptoms get worse, or you begin to feel like a cripple, see a doctor.

FINGER INJURIES

A player who hasn't jammed a finger during a baseball game probably just wasn't trying very hard. It's a remarkably easy thing to do, and it can also make you miserable. Most often, though, it's not a serious problem. Your finger will hurt, it may get stiff and swollen, it may turn black and blue. Ice will make the pain more bearable. Don't let anyone talk you into popping the finger. If it's whacked way out of line, you should see a doctor. A badly jammed finger can take six months or even longer to get full motion back. In the meantime, when you play, tape the jammed finger to an adjoining healthy finger for support.

A baseball or mallet finger is more serious than the usual jammed finger. It occurs in the same way—during a bad catch, usually—but it involves the distal joint, or tip, of the finger. Either the extensor tendon is torn away from its attachment to the bone, or the bone itself has been pulled loose. Either way, the tip of the finger droops and you can't actively straighten it. If that's your situation, you should see a doctor. A permanent droop or worse may be the result if you ignore it. The required treatment is to put your finger in a splint. It will have to stay there constantly for six weeks. Don't risk trouble by taking it off sooner.

SHOULDER SEPARATION

A particular affliction of baseball, softball and hockey players is known as an acromio-clavicular separation. It's what goes wrong when a ballplayer dives for a flyball and lands on the point of his shoulder, driving it down and tearing the ligaments that hold the clavicle in place against the acromion. If the tear is complete, the player comes up with a clavicle sticking out like—well, like a sore thumb, only it hurts a lot more. And when he tries to move the shoulder it will hurt and feel tender, too. This is not a self-treatable injury. You'll need to see a doctor.

SLIDING—A NECESSARY EVIL

The experts agree: when in doubt, slide, and when in trouble, slide hard. The best way to slide is a subject of some debate. A headfirst slide toward home plate is never appropriate; you could wind up with a mouthful of shin guards. And you could get spiked on the fingers or hand if you're not careful. On the other bases, if you slide in headfirst you stand less of a chance of breaking a leg or ripping up an ankle. The worst kind of slide is the one that comes out of indecision. If you're going to get spiked, practically speaking, a hand will heal faster than an ankle. If you're going to slide, do it with everything you've got, and then some. A good slide can mean extra bases; it can also mean a nasty abrasion, some ugly bruises or a sprained ankle. Chapter 4 tells how to treat such minor injuries.

GETTING BACK INTO THE GAME

Sitting on the sidelines after you've been injured is frustrating. Worse still, though, is injuring yourself all over again. So give your body a chance to heal fully before throwing yourself back into competition. Return to play when you can make all the moves—throwing, running, hitting, stop-starting, chasing—normally. A serious sprain may keep you out for a month; a pulled shoulder muscle may heal in a few days. When an ankle sprain is severe enough to require a cast, you'll need to rehabilitate it totally before returning to the field. Don't try to play without a full functional recovery. If you do, the problem can become chronic. A badly sprained ankle that isn't immobilized until it's fully healed can become the ankle that gives out on you when you least expect it. A single pebble can bring a great player down, if his ankle is acting up.

IV. Know Your Body, Prevent Your Injuries

16. Hot Spots: A Body

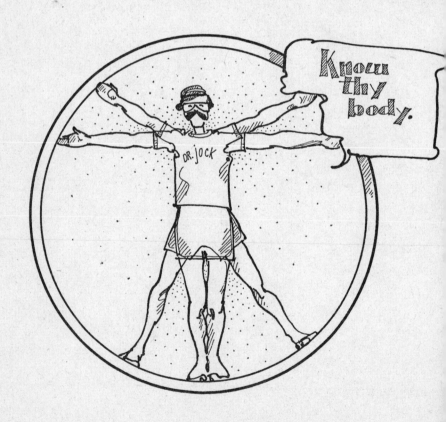

Owner's Manual

The more you know about your body, the more familiar you are with the names of all the places that can get hurt, the better off you are. It's awfully easy to remain alienated from your body, to think of *it* as somehow separate from *you*. But your own unhurried moves toward fitness will have made you more aware of your body, yourself, than ever before. Your body is, after all, the sum total of all its moving parts and when a whole group of them unite in painful chorus to declare that your knee is so sore you'll have to give up exercising, then you ought to be curious about what has gone wrong.

To help you do this, we'll begin by identifying the body parts and places where you're most likely to have trouble, and the specific things that can go wrong, so that you can decide whether the injury is one you can most likely handle on your own, or had better see a doctor for.

The chart on page 262 should help. You can use this chart if you are in the grip of some grievous pain. Find your sport, find your hot spot and follow your finger to the top of the chart where we've listed the page number you can turn to for fast help.

THE FOOT

Take a look at the diagram of the foot, with its complex network of ligaments and bones, all precisely sculpted and aligned for maximum support. That's what the foot is really for: support. The central feature in that whole support system is the arch. The arch of the human foot evolved as the species evolved toward standing upright. It's a clever innovation, really, since an arch will support and distribute weight much more efficiently than a flat surface. The Romans picked up on nature's structural discovery when they started building temples with vaulted roofs.

If your arch isn't up to the ideal building code, if it's too high or too flat, so that any of your bones are even slightly out of line, you are

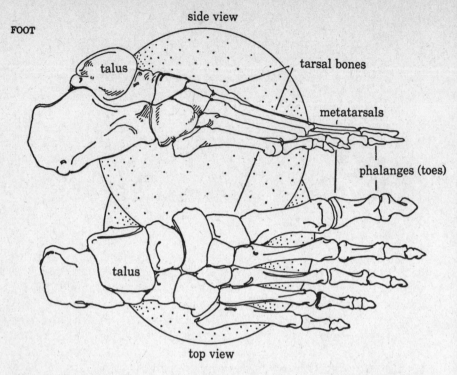

FOOT

side view

talus

tarsal bones

metatarsals

phalanges (toes)

talus

top view

going to have trouble with your feet. Runners are especially likely to suffer foot problems because for every mile they run, they pound each foot into the ground 800 times. All this stress and pounding can take, and will take, its toll if you're not aware of some basic foot care.

BUY THE BEST SHOES YOU CAN

Poorly constructed, ill-fitting shoes are no bargain. They can cause you a lot of grief in a running sport, and if you're having trouble with a strained arch, a heel spur or a tendinitis, the first thing to check is your shoes. The athletic shoe business is big business now, and for the most part the better specialty shoes are designed to meet all the basic requirements in terms of cushioning and support. Of course, there are differences—and these are gone into from time to time by the running magazines and various consumer guides—but when it comes to buying a good shoe, all the expert opinion in the world can't determine which pair of shoes fits your particular foot, and best supports your arch. Your Number 1 shoe may be someone else's Number 3. The important thing is to get a shoe that gives your foot stability and allows flexibility with enough cushion to ease the pounding. When you try it on for fit, you should have on the same combination of socks you'll use in running. Tell the salesperson what sort of surface you run on; some shoes are designed for soft surfaces, others for hard. Sometimes you come up with the best fitting shoe only after trial and error, and sometimes you can run through five or six different kinds and still have foot problems. That is frequently when you have to turn to orthotics.

ORTHOTICS CAN BE HELPFUL

An orthotic is a special appliance that fits inside your athletic shoe and supports your foot as you run and move about. More and more runners are turning to orthotics to correct the causes of foot pain. Making them to fit your foot and suit your needs exactly is a precision business, best left to experts. Sometimes you can get relief from a commercially available orthotic (Scholl's #610, for instance), and you'd be wise to try it since the ones you buy over the counter are much less expensive than those that are custom-made. But if you're still hurting, you'll have to go to an orthopedic specialist or a podiatrist and have one made. This can be expensive—$150 or more—but it's still a bargain if it gives you relief. If you possibly can, deal with a doctor or a podiatrist who has some interest and experience in sports medicine. The more patients that have come before you with similar problems, the better your treatment is bound to be.

STRESS FRACTURES

You're running along and all of a sudden, out of the blue, you feel a sharp pain in your foot. The pain is so bad you have to stop. In the next couple of days your foot swells up and gets red and tender. You rest, you do your deep breathing exercises, you try and fantasize the pain away. You go for an X-ray and it doesn't show a thing. Still, no matter how hard you try, you can't get back to running. But when you go back to your doctor three weeks later, he is finally able to make a diagnosis. What you have is a stress fracture—a hairline crack in one wall or cortex of the bone. Runners frequently get them in the metatarsals or the tibia, probably because their feet are in poor condition, and they've tried to push themselves too far, too soon. The crack may be so small that it doesn't show up, but your doctor can spot the new bone that is laid down to heal it.

If you get a stress fracture, you'll be off your running feet for at least six weeks. You won't need a cast, and a good firm shoe will allow you to walk on it. When you do get back to running, start out slowly to recondition yourself, or you can expect another stress fracture somewhere down the line.

HEEL AND ARCH PROBLEMS

It's not fair to be cursed with flat feet or a high arch, but it is common. The arch of the foot is maintained by the bony architecture and a tough, fibrous band called the plantar fascia, which runs from the metatarsal heads (the anatomist's name for the ball of your foot) to the calcaneus, or heel bone. The heel spur that you may see on an X-ray photograph is really the attachment of the plantar fascia to the bone. It always points up and forward on the calcaneus, never down into the heel. When you run, your arch spreads a bit under pressure every time you take a step and land. The more pressure, the more spread is needed to absorb it. This spreading stretches the plantar fascia. When this happens too often to an unconditioned foot, when wearing a shoe that doesn't give enough support or cushioning, or when there is too frequent running on a hard, unbending surface, this ligament or its attachment to the bone can be strained. If you do that, it will hurt. If your calf muscle is too tight, you'll put even more strain on this structure. So one thing to do if your heel hurts is to work on your calf muscles for flexibility. You can also cut down a bit on your distance until the pain subsides. If the problem persists, you can use a special arch support, a heel cup or pad to cushion the blow. To ease the pain, use ice on your heel after running, and take aspirin. If the pain is so intense that you can't walk, you might see your doctor about a possible injection of hydrocortisone, keeping in mind that cortisone can have nasty side effects. You're better off in a program that forestalls the pain instead of camouflaging it. Some doctors may spot that heel spur and advise having it surgically removed. David has never found that necessary or even helpful, since the bone spur points up into the foot and doesn't seem to be the cause of the pain.

Another kind of heel pain common among runners comes from wearing too-thin track shoes. The less cushioning you have, the more likely you are to bruise the fat pad in your heel against a rock or hard spot. This fat pad is a specialized structure, consisting of a lot of compartments separated by bands of fibrous tissue to help maintain it. If you get a hematoma here, a bad bruise, it will take some time for your body to deal with it. While it is healing, use ice to relieve the pain. Don't keep pounding on it—you'll just prolong the problem.

JOGGER'S TOE (SAME AS TENNIS TOE)

Remember the last time you took off your sock after running 12 miles in new shoes and discovered an ugly accumulation of blood under your toenail? That's jogger's toe, a common complaint of runners and cross-country skiers. It happens because your toes jam against a too-tight shoe or (less frequently) a too-tight sock. To correct or avoid this, make sure your shoes are designed with ample room in the toe box, and wear enough comfortable socks to cushion the toes. Jogger's toe may turn your nail black and blue and look awful, but it's not very serious. It's not even especially painful, and even if you eventually lose the nail, you have nothing much to worry about. The bruise will heal naturally. If it feels tender, put a Band-Aid around it for a couple of days.

BLISTERS

Some of the biggest, strongest jocks we know have been brought whimpering to their knees because of simple blisters. This is a heat injury to the skin produced by friction. The cells burst, fluid accumulates, the area is tender and quite painful. You can prevent blisters by toughening your skin gradually, but this takes time and patience. In the meantime, do whatever you can to reduce friction on your feet. Don't wear shoes that are too big or too small. If you wear socks, smooth out any wrinkles before you put your shoes on. Sometimes wearing two pairs of socks can help increase sliding, thus reducing friction. It's also important that you keep your feet as dry as possible. Moisture increases friction. Powder sprinkled in your shoe and on your feet can help, and if you tend to sweat a lot, you should carry a dry pair of socks to change into.

As soon as you feel a hot spot developing on your foot, stop and take care of it. Don't wait for a blister to develop. Dry your feet with powder or use a lubricant jelly covered with a Band-Aid or moleskin padding. If you do get a blister, you'll see a blob of skin filled with fluid. *Don't burst it.* Intact skin is your best barrier against infection. Calvin Coolidge's son actually died from an infection a couple of days after he got a blister playing tennis. If the bleb is too big and too painful to ignore, you can let some of the fluid out by sterilizing a needle and gently draining the blister. Avoid popping or shredding it. If it does tear, cleanse it thoroughly with soap and water and cover it with a sterile dressing. You'd be smart to stay away from running on it until it heals.

THE ANKLE

Most ankle problems are due to injuries: a sprain or a fracture. If you're a runner, though, it is possible to develop pain on the outside of the ankle. This happens because, for one reason or another, the foot constantly gives in each time you land, causing undue stress and strain on the inside ligaments and pinching the joint lining on the outside. Check the bottom of your running shoe and see whether you're wearing down one side more than the other. Ideally, the pattern of wear ought to be even. If it's not, you might try to correct your running form, or you may want to see a specialist about an orthotic.

Ankle injuries are common in all sports. Volleyball players can trip over rocks, baseball players may slide wrong, tennis players may stumble over a loose ball. The ankle itself is a very complicated

ANKLE

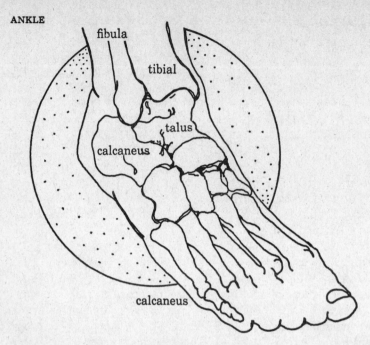

fibula

tibial

talus

calcaneus

calcaneus

mechanism, designed to bear more body weight than any other joint. It is held in place, to simplify, by its bony architecture and by a complex set of ligaments that connect the three bones of the ankle joint to one another, and to all the bones in the foot. The system is strong but it's also vulnerable, and if you're not careful, you can wind up with a serious, debilitating injury.

ANKLE SPRAIN

A sprain is actually a tearing of the ligaments. Most often it occurs on the outside of the ankle, where the ligaments aren't as strong as on the inside. Ankle sprains can be classified as mild, moderate or severe. If you have a severe one, you'll know it because the pain will be intense, and you'll want to get to a doctor as soon as you can. A severe sprain means you've torn one or more of the three ligaments on the outside of your ankle. This will leave you in a very unstable condition, and you'll need to lug a cast around for anywhere from four to six weeks. If you leave it untreated, you'll end up with a chronic problem, an ankle that gives way at the slightest misstep. Sometimes, if there is continuing instability, the only answer is surgery.

A mild ankle sprain is one you can self-treat. Sure, it hurts at the time, so that your first thought is to hobble to an emergency room, but the severe pain subsides in a while. If you are able to move it through a full range of motion, you can probably take care of it yourself. You must expect some swelling and some black-and-blue discoloration.

Tearing a ligament, even just a few fibers, causes internal bleeding, and bleeding causes pain, swelling and bruises. Get some ice on the ankle, wrap it with an elastic bandage and elevate it, higher than your hip.

After an ankle injury, you should return to play only when you've regained full functional use. If you can't stop and start, shift and twist, without pain, you don't belong back in the game. If you return to activity too fast, you will reinjure your ankle and maybe make it worse.

Chronically weak ankles can be a problem, and we're always hearing from athletes who want to learn how to strengthen their ankles. Sorry, but it's not possible. Your ankle is primarily bone and ligament and you can't strengthen either of those. You can, however, strengthen the muscles that control the ankle, such as the calf muscle and the anterior tibial muscle. Chapter 8 tells you how to do that.

Wrapping your ankle may also help a delicate situation somewhat; we've shown you how to do that in Chapter 4. When you apply an elastic bandage, just roll it on, don't stretch it. Some swelling will occur naturally, and rolling the bandage on will let that happen without making the bandage too tight. If it does become too tight, the pain will become worse, there may be some numbness, and instead of their normal pink, the toes will have a bluish tinge. Don't be alarmed, though, if the ankle, foot and toes become black and blue, or if the discoloration spreads up into the lower leg. That's normal.

LATERAL ANKLE PAIN

Runners with flat or overflexible arches can wind up with pain just in front of, or below, the bone on the outside of the ankle. This comes from an alignment problem; since the foot turns in with every flat-footed step, the joint lining on the outside gets pinched, and that hurts. A good solid running shoe will usually prevent this problem. If it develops anyhow, you'll have to see an orthopedist or podiatrist interested in sports medicine for a custom-fitted orthotic.

ANKLE FRACTURES

An ankle can snap, crackle and pop pretty easily, so if you take a serious fall, or if you hear something give way on your way down, you'd better have an X-ray. If you've broken a bone you can expect to be off your game for at least six weeks. How quickly you can return to it is directly related to how willing you are to work at it.

THE LOWER LEGS

Between your ankle and your knee a lot of things can go wrong, but we're going to deal with the three most common complaints: shin splints, calf muscle tears and a ruptured or inflamed Achilles tendon.

SHIN SPLINTS

This is not the name of any specific ailment, but simply a catchall term for any kind of pain you feel in the front of the leg between the knee and the ankle. If you have that kind of pain and it won't go away, you should see a doctor for diagnosis and treatment.

When this kind of pain hits you on the outside of the leg, it is called the anterior compartment syndrome. It is caused by overuse—too much, too soon—and it most often strikes runners and cross-country skiers. The muscles in the anterior compartment are the ones responsible for pulling your foot up. If they are undertrained and overstrained, they will start to swell. That means they will hurt. Stopping the exercise usually relieves the symptoms. Ice will help, too. On rare occasions, when the swelling is very great, this can develop into a serious problem. Since the muscles are enclosed in a tight compartment, one or more of them can die, literally strangled to death by the swelling. If you have pain on the outside of your lower leg that keeps getting worse, even with ice applications, don't wait about seeing your doctor.

You can prevent this problem by gradual training and working on flexibility. If your calf muscles are too tight, the anterior muscles will have to work harder. Changing to a softer running or playing surface will sometimes help too.

Pain on the inner side of your lower leg can be tough to diagnose. Several things can cause it. It's usually due to overuse, and a tendency toward flat-footedness aggravates the problem. The posterior tibial muscle and tendon start in the back of your leg, run behind your ankle bone and attach to the inside of your foot. They enable you to turn your foot in and help support the arch. However, if you run so that your foot rolls in each time you land, you may strain that muscle. When that happens, you are a candidate for posterior tibial tendinitis. (This may be felt at the place where the tendon attaches on the inside of your foot, rather than in your leg.)

If the situation is chronic, you may pull away the muscle attachment from the bone—a disorder called periostitis. This causes pain and tenderness along the inside of the tibia.

Another injury with similar symptoms occurs when constant pull on the inside of the bone causes a stress fracture of the tibia. Then the bone is literally pulled apart.

If you are flat-footed, the force on the inside of your leg is increased, and your chances of suffering one of these shin-splint injuries is increased. An abnormal running gait can also bring them on (e.g., when your leg lands too close to the midline of your body) and so can running on a curved track, the same way, all the time. If you run on a curved track and are having lower leg problems, you can try switching directions. Running shoes with good arch supports will help prevent these problems. So will proper conditioning. If you do develop the symptoms, you'd better see a doctor. You'll need an X-ray and you may need a special orthotic. Using ice at home, on your own, will help relieve the symptomatic pain.

If the X-ray shows you have a stress fracture—and that's not as uncommon among runners as you might think—you'll have to wait until it heals before you return to running or sports. That could mean a minimum of six weeks off. If your diagnosis is periostitis, you may be helped by the anti-inflammatory drug, Butazolidin. You can run with it so long as you stay at a comfortable pace and avoid hard surfaces.

CALF MUSCLE AND ACHILLES TENDON INJURIES

Both of these lower-leg ailments are painfully common in all sports that require a lot of running around, especially among once-or-twice-a-week players who do a lot of quick starts and stops but don't exercise often enough to really get into condition.

Calf muscle tears are due to inflexibility. If the muscle is inelastic, it can tear when it is suddenly put under stress. When that happens, or when the Achilles tendon rips, the pain is sharp and sudden, and may ground you. It feels as though something has snapped, or as though someone had taken a tennis racquet and whacked you on the back of the leg. You know right away that you're in trouble.

Partial tears of the calf muscle occur on the inside of the calf, at the fleshy part. If you've pulled a calf muscle, you'll be able to locate a tender spot. You can expect it to be swollen the next day, and in a few days it will be black and blue. You will find it painful to try to stand on tiptoes. To treat it, use the standard first-aid measures: Ice, Compression, Elevation (see Chapter 4). Wearing a shoe with an elevated heel can relieve some of the pain by taking the pressure off the muscle. If it hurts a lot, you may need crutches or a cane for a few days. You should see a doctor to verify your own diagnosis, and you can expect to be out of sorts and out of sports for about six weeks. Before you return to full activity, you'll have to work hard to restore flexibility and strength. Start with wall leans to stretch the calf, and progress to toe raises with weights to make it strong.

Achilles tendon tears require professional treatment—either surgery or a cast.

THE KNEE

The knee is the most injured and least understood joint in sports. It withstands incredible stresses from twists and turns, leaps and bounces. You can pound it for miles and miles and it keeps coming back for more. But sometimes it breaks down, if the forces are too great, the stress too much. Let one little thing go wrong and you can end up with a swollen, painful knee that could plague you forever.

EVERYONE IS VULNERABLE

Runners and jumpers, skiers and tennis players, all athletes who use their legs risk knee problems. You can get tendinitis from overuse—too much stress, too often. Runners and swimmers may get mild but irritating ligament sprains on the inside or the outside of the knee,

KNEE JOINT

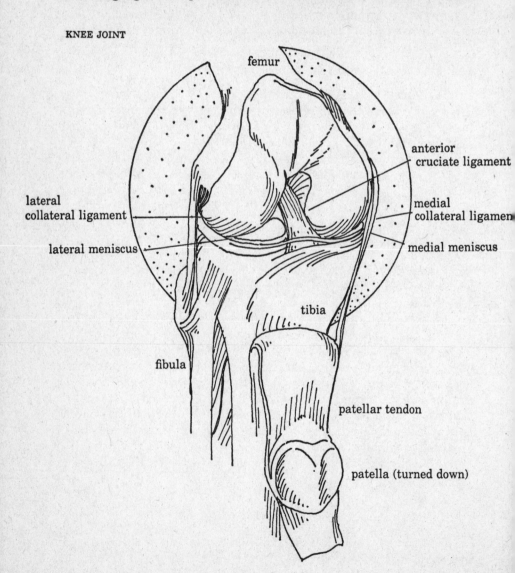

caused by variations in foot or leg alignment. Falls by skiers wearing the new higher boots take their toll on the knee, and so do collision sports—rugby, soccer and football. Especially football. The knee just isn't built for such rough action. Cartilages can tear anytime they're caught between the rotating bones of the knee, particularly if the knee is bent and the foot is fixed. Falls on the knee can damage the joint surface, particularly the patella or kneecap. Women athletes who have a tendency to be knock-kneed (male athletes tend more toward being bow-legged) have special problems with chondromalacia, the steady eroding of the underside of the kneecap, and dislocating kneecaps.

Why is everyone so vulnerable? Because the knee is the most complex joint in the body. Not only does it bend and straighten like a hinge, it also rotates as it extends. This rotating action locks the knee and makes standing easier, but it means that we can't make a knee brace that is strong enough to support the knee and, at the same time, flexible enough to accommodate the rotation.

Once you have a clear understanding of the knee's complexity, perhaps you'll take a little more time keeping it strong and flexible. As the rounded ends of the femur (the upper leg bone) move on the flatter top of the tibia (the lower leg bone), they both hinge and slide. Those cartilages or menisci that cause so much trouble both help to stabilize the joint as it moves back and forth, and help cushion it against some of the shocks that are given to it. The radius of motion is not the same at the front of the joint as it is in the back, since the condyles, the ends of the femur, are not concentric. The ligaments that hold the joint together, from side to side and from front to back, must work at different lengths as the joint moves. All these conditions must be met for your knee to work normally; moreover, the surfaces of the joint itself must remain perfectly smooth and intact to reduce friction as the knee moves.

With all of this going on at once, it's no wonder there are so many knee troubles. Diagnosis is difficult because there *are* so many things that can go wrong. Almost anytime something does, there is swelling in the knee. This means that the joint lining is irritated, causing fluid to build up there—causing "water on the knee," which makes diagnosis even more difficult.

Any knee that remains painful or swollen after an injury should be checked by a responsible doctor, preferably one who is geared to sports medicine. If you didn't suffer a blow or an injury and your knee got sore all by itself, it will most likely heal all by itself, the way tendinitis does. But you should find out the cause of the problem so that you can take some positive action to either remedy it or prevent it from happening again. If your knee pain is due to chronic ligament strain, an orthotic in your shoe may save you. But knee pain from chondromalacia is a different story entirely, and it won't go away by itself no matter how long you rest.

PATELLAR TENDINITIS

Pain around the knee seems to be the Number 1 complaint of runners. The causes are legion, but one of the most common is patellar tendinitis, or jumper's knee. Basketball and volleyball players get it too. The patellar tendon attaches to the inferior tip of the kneecap. (Sometimes the problem occurs at the top of the kneecap in the attachment of the quadriceps tendon.) Like all tendinitis, this is an overuse syndrome: too much use for too long, with too little flexibility and conditioning. If your quadriceps muscle is tight and inflexible, too much tension is placed on the patellar tendon and small tears eventually occur. After a while, you'll begin to feel it. You may experience a sharp stab of pain at the knee when you run, especially on hills, or you may feel it in climbing stairs or squatting. It might show up as a dull, aggravating ache after you've sat in one position for a long time, and a sharp pain when you get up. The only tender spot will be under the tip of the knee, and your doctor will have to tip up the kneecap to find it. Occasionally, the knee will feel squeaky over the tendon when you rub it, but that usually happens only when the condition is severe. The discomfort comes from swelling in the tendon, which may not be visible on the outside, but is still enough to cause considerable pain.

What can you do if you get it? The important thing to know is that if you develop patellar tendinitis, you can continue to play your sport without worrying about doing more damage to your knee. As in all tendinitis, the body will eventually heal itself. The healing process can be slow, however. It may take a year or more. Meanwhile, if you can overcome the pain enough to enjoy your sport, by all means continue it. And there are some things you can do to relieve some of the symptoms.

Before you work out, heat up your knee with warm water or a heating pad, and make sure that you take time to fully stretch the quads and hamstrings. After your workout, wrap a plastic bag of ice around your knee to cut down swelling and pain. If you need to, continue this 3 or 4 times a day, 15 minutes a session, for the next day or two. A rounded or cushioned heel might help by taking some of the strain off the tendon, too. Aspirin also will help reduce the inflammation.

Deal with the pain as best you can, using deep breathing, relaxation, visualization—whatever works for you. If you can't cope, by all means see a doctor. But an injection of hydrocortisone into your patellar tendon is to be avoided. Hydrocortisone shots will alter the structure of the tendon, and repeated shots, with the pain masked, may cause the patellar tendon to rupture. Then you're really in trouble. Experienced sports physicians may try one small shot (¼ ml), just once to help acute cases.

What about surgery? It's true that some professional athletes have had operations for this problem (David did one on Tom Boerwinkle's knee, to drop just one Bull's name). Since their livelihood depends on being able to play ball, the pros feel that they can't afford to wait out Mother Nature on the bench, allowing the year or more the injury may need to heal by itself. But youngsters and recreational athletes who develop this problem are probably better off without surgery. If it hurts too much for you to carry on your sport, switch to swimming or cycling to keep fit while your knee is healing. When you do get back into action, you'll have to follow a slow comeback program of strengthening and flexibility.

PATELLAR TENDON RUPTURE

Sudden, violent jumping can sometimes lead to ruptures of the patellar or quadriceps tendon, above or below the kneecap. This happens more to basketball and volleyball players than to other athletes, and when it does happen, the injury is sudden and severe. You jump, and when you come down, your knee buckles. It could have torn when you jumped or when you landed; either way, you can't straighten your leg, lift it or stand. If you put your finger where it hurts, you'll find a hole where the tendon was. This injury requires an operation, a cast for six to eight weeks and a long program of supervised physical therapy. It's not the kind of rehabilitation program you can do in your own home—you'll need experts around to show you exactly what to do and how to do it. These tendons won't rupture unless for some reason they are already abnormal. You can help yourself avoid the problem by making sure your quadriceps muscle is strong and stretched before you jump around on it.

PATELLAR DISLOCATION

Women athletes have one problem that is largely peculiar to them. That is repeated dislocations, partial or complete, of the kneecap. It happens to women more than to men because women tend to be knock-kneed (the result of having a wider pelvis to accommodate the birth canal). Because of being knock-kneed, the quadriceps tends to pull the kneecap to the outside. If the muscles on the inside of the kneecap are weak, particularly the vastus medialis just above and on the inside of the kneecap, the patella can be pulled off track and out of place when the quadriceps suddenly contracts.

What happens then? It hurts and you fall down. Often, when you straighten your knee, the kneecap will snap back into place. If it doesn't and is hung up somehow, you'll have to have it put back by a doctor. If it goes on popping out repeatedly, you may require surgery to realign the attachment; but at first it can be handled more conservatively.

If you've torn some of the muscle attachments on the inside of the kneecap, you'll probably need a cast for anywhere from four to six weeks to hold it immobile while it heals. Before you can get back into action, you'll have to rehabilitate your knee, concentrating particularly on strengthening the vastus medialis muscle that helps keep the kneecap in place. You'll find a good exercise for that in the section on chondromalacia.

OSGOOD-SCHLATTER SYNDROME

This is not a running injury—though it is often mistaken for one—but a syndrome that affects growing children. If you're a 12-year-old with knee pain, or the worried parent of a youngster who complains that his knee hurts every time he plays basketball, you should understand what might be going on.

The Osgood-Schlatter syndrome affects the growth center where the patellar tendon attaches to the tibia. No one knows the cause, but apparently there is a temporary loss of blood supply to the tendon attachment. This is not an injury but a condition, and the good news is that it will go away in time. Meanwhile, you can expect to see a bump that is tender to the touch. The knee feels worse when you climb stairs, get up from a chair, or run or jump. It isn't dangerous and the pain will go away when growth is complete and the growth center fuses to the rest of the bone. Although playing ball and running around can make it hurt, you won't be doing your body any harm. You can continue to do whatever you feel like doing, so long as the pain doesn't get so bad that it takes away all the fun.

You generally don't need any treatment other than heat on the knee before you play, and ice afterward. If the pain gets to the point where you can't walk, a cast extending from the ankle to the top of the thigh for four to six weeks should give relief. There is no evidence that this will cause the bone to break, nor is there any indication that surgery is necessary.

CHONDROMALACIA

This common knee problem involves roughness on the underside of the kneecap, and is really a form of arthritis that comes from the gradual wearing away of the joint surface. Heredity naturally plays some part, but the degenerative process can start following an injury—such as encountering a 260-pound tackle on the 27-yard line—or it can start with a dislocation. Sometimes it begins to wear down because the quadriceps muscle isn't lined up properly and the patella rides to the outside of the groove and wears out. You may be susceptible, too, if you are knock-kneed or your tibia rotates out too far. If you are flat-footed and you run without proper arch support, the knee tends to go in when you land and the quadriceps pulls the kneecap out—also a process that causes excessive wear.

Some people have inadequate muscle on the inside of the thigh—the vastus medialis, the muscle just above and on the inside of the kneecap, which controls the position of the patella as it glides through the groove at the end of the femur. If the muscle is weak, the patella rides to the outside and wears out.

Doing bend-and-straighten knee extension exercises with weights will aggravate the situation (though some teams and trainers persist in prescribing them), particularly after a knee operation or an injury where there is still some fluid in the knee.

The major symptoms will be pain when you move your knee. If it is bad enough or goes on long enough, there will be some swelling. This is because fragments of the articular surface break off and act as mechanical irritants to the joint lining, causing synovitis (inflammation of the synovial membrane). With inflammation, there may also be atrophy of the thigh muscles, especially the vastus medialis. Since this controls the position of the patella, weak and atrophied muscles only aggravate the situation. Then you've got a vicious cycle: pain, inflammation, weakness, wear; more pain, inflammation, weakness, wear and so on.

So what do you do for chondromalacia? First, you see a responsible doctor, preferably one who has seen enough such cases to make a proper diagnosis and who is geared toward getting you active again as soon as possible. If you're a runner, tell the doctor that and make sure he conducts his examination with your pants off and both your legs bare. (As you can see from our explanation, a lot of things in and about your legs can contribute to chondromalacia, and he can't see the whole picture with your jeans rolled up over your knee and your shoes and socks on.)

Treatment should be aimed at cutting down the inflammation (ice, aspirin, maybe some anti-inflammatory medication) and restoring the strength to your leg muscles. (Chapter 8 gives strengthening exercises for the knees.) Choose your rehabilitation program carefully: doing knee extensions with weights may make matters worse, and step-ups are equally irritating to the kneecap.

An excellent exercise for this condition is an isometric one aimed at strengthening the vastus medialis. Done properly, it will help build the kneecap-stabilizing muscle where you need it most without wearing out the undersurface of the kneecap. To do it, lie flat on your back with your knees straight. Stick your ankle under a heavy desk, or some other immovable object, with a towel folded over the ankle to pad it. Tighten your anterior thigh muscles (the quadriceps), keep your knee straight, and try to lift your leg up against the resistance that you can't actually move. Contract the muscle, and really press hard. Hold the position for 5 seconds and relax. Repeat this 5 times. Do this routine at least once a day; twice a day is even better.

What about elastic wraps and those slip-on bandages that completely cover the knee? In general, we would say that they only make things worse, since they push the kneecap against the femur. However, the kind with a cutout to take pressure off the patella, and a pad to hold it in place, might help.

Prevention of chondromalacia is tricky. You can try to avoid blows and falls, and you should keep your leg muscles strong so that your kneecap will be stable; but if you have a tendency toward developing it, as with arthritis, there's not much you can do about it. Once your doctor has made the diagnosis, it is probable that it will slowly get worse.

Chondromalacia is not one of those ailments that allow you to tough it out and keep on playing. Repeated bent-knee, weight-bearing exercise (such as running) will usually aggravate it, so you may have to look around for another fitness sport, such as swimming, that takes the pressure off the knee.

If you have a lot of swelling, your knee may have to be drained of fluid (aspirated). An injection of cortisone is a possibility, but only as a last resort—and only with the understanding that the drug can alter the chemical structure of the articular cartilage and shouldn't be done more than two or three times.

A new technique, using an arthroscope to thoroughly flush out the debris inside the joint, can give fairly long-lasting, though still temporary, relief. If the disability is severe, it may call for surgery. Hopefully, the problem can be treated by debridement, shaving down the rough surfaces, but if not, you are left with two choices: patellectomy or patellar replacement.

Most surgeons remove the kneecap—a patellectomy. You can function well without the kneecap, but you will need to work hard at rehabilitating the leg muscles that normally surround it. You won't lose the ability to bend your knee fully, but you will lose some strength because the main function of the kneecap is to act as a fulcrum for your quadriceps muscle.

The second choice is to replace the worn-out kneecap with an artificial one, but David is not enthusiastic about this. Artificial kneecaps certainly aren't meant to take the stresses and strains of most sports. You can work your way back to running after you've had a patellectomy but if you've had it replaced, you don't stand a chance.

KNEE CARTILAGE INJURIES

Let's say your toes are planted firmly on the baseline and you're waiting for the tennis ball. Suddenly you see it come whizzing by you to the left, and you quickly twist your torso, hoping to catch enough of it to make a return. Then—whammo!—you feel a sharp pain in your knee and hear a click that tells you something bad has happened. You've probably torn the cartilage by trapping it as you twist. Since a routine X-ray won't show torn cartilage, making a diagnosis is not a simple matter; arthrograms (a series of X-rays taken of a joint in various positions following an injection of dye and/or air) and arthroscopy (performed by an instrument inserted directly into the joint) will help considerably.

Cartilage injuries show up in several ways. If your knee is locked, the diagnosis is simple: you'll need surgery. A locked knee, one that can't be moved through a full range of motion, won't heal properly by itself. Another sign of injury to the cartilage is swelling, but that's common to practically all knee problems. You can help in making the diagnosis by being aware of how your knee feels: does it seem to buckle or give way when you walk? Did you hear a click when you lunged to the left? Another tip-off that something major has happened to a knee is atrophy, the shrinking or wasting of the muscles around it. This is usually the result of a serious injury to the knee.

A torn cartilage is a foreign body inside the knee joint, and every time it catches or is pinched there, it can do damage to the joint surface. It will need to be removed before it does permanent damage. But when cartilage is removed you've lost something you need, and the knee will never be the same. You can work your way back to sports and continue a healthy, active life, but this will take time, sweat and determination on your part. If the surgery is solely for a cartilage tear, you should not need a cast. You will need a formal physical therapy program, however, one prescribed by your doctor and religiously practiced by yourself. If you can afford a physical therapist, go see one; your recovery will be faster if you're supervised. The fastest possible recovery will take about six weeks, and, for most people, two or three months is more likely. Make no mistake about it: it is hard work to get back into playing shape, but the alternative is worse.

KNEE LIGAMENT INJURIES

An athlete with a torn knee ligament has a serious injury. It usually results from severe trauma such as a clipping injury in football or a high speed twist over a fixed foot in a skiing fall. Almost all these injuries are felt on the inside of the knee. These severe injuries may involve more than one ligament in the knee. With these injuries, you usually know that something serious has happened, and don't need encouragement to see a doctor. Occasionally, with single ligament injuries, the initial pain may subside and allow you to remain active for a few hours. Eventually, though, pain and swelling will force you to seek medical advice. Incomplete tears need protection so that they don't become complete tears, and complete tears require surgery.

Injured collateral ligaments can be repaired with surgery, but the cruciate ligaments—so called because they cross over each other like an X—cannot. They will have to be substituted for, and even the best surgical operation leaves your knee less stable than before the injury. The final outcome will be only as good as your determination and ability to rehabilitate your knee. The tear may take two seconds, the surgery two hours; but proper rehabilitation could take a year. You can expect to be in a cast for about six weeks after this kind of surgery.

COLLATERAL LIGAMENT STRAINS

The collateral ligaments keep your knee from moving too far from side to side. Like all ligaments, they can sprain under pressure. If your leg or foot isn't properly aligned, or you have a high-arched foot with the heel turned in, your knee naturally thrusts out every time you land. With your foot landing about 800 times every mile you run, it won't take long to strain either the lateral collateral ligament, on the outside of your knee, or the iliotibial band, the tight band of tissue that you can feel running down the outside of your knee. If you run flat-footed, your knee thrusts in as you land and you can strain the medial collateral ligament on the inside of your knee. In all these instances you will feel a burning pain as you run and you may have a persistent ache afterward, caused by swelling. Ice should help. Training gradually, with a slow build-up of mileage, and avoiding overuse, will usually prevent problems when the variation is minor. If your malalignment is major, however, a well-made, properly fitted orthotic may allow you to go on running. Cut back the distance you run to the point where you are free of pain, and wait for the ligaments to heal.

HAMSTRINGS

The hamstrings are the primary knee flexors that stretch along the back of the thigh, and athletes of every description frequently injure them. And yet such injuries are nearly always avoidable. Although the hamstrings become strong and tight in running, runners frequently injure them because they are not kept as flexible as they should be. When push comes to stretch, the hamstrings simply can't take it. Basketball, baseball, football and soccer require the players to make sudden changes of speed and length of stride. If the hamstrings are weak or inflexible, the force of these sudden shifts may be more than the muscle can stand, so it is torn.

The more flexible you are, the more likely it is that the tearing will be minor. When it does happen you will usually feel a sharp pain in the back of the thigh, anywhere from the pelvis to the knee. You won't be able to continue playing, and it may get worse the next day because of the bleeding and swelling. After a few days there may be black-and-blue discoloration. If you're injured this way, don't try to tough it out; you'll only make a bad situation worse. Stop playing, apply ice and roll on a 6-inch elastic bandage around your thigh. If the pain gets so bad that you can't walk, see a doctor. You may need crutches for a while.

How fast you recover from a pulled hamstring depends on how badly you've been hurt, and how willing you are to work on getting back your flexibility and strength. The process may well take six weeks. While you recover, you should use ice to reduce swelling, and concentrate first on stretching. Do not push to the point of pain, just to the point of pull. Once you have regained flexibility in your hamstring, you can work on strength. Your hamstrings will never be as strong as your quadriceps, nor should they be, but you'll need to regain full function, so that the injured leg is equal to the uninjured leg, if you hope to get back to sports and not reinjure yourself.

Remember to reintroduce your hamstring to stress slowly. If you're a runner, don't think you can run the distance you ran before your injury. Build slowly, or you risk painful, crippling reinjury. In the meantime, while you are waiting for your hamstring to heal, you don't have to sit around and mope about your poor condition. You probably can swim or ride a bicycle to keep in shape.

GROIN PULLS

Groin pulls are another common sports injury, similar to a hamstring pull and just as avoidable. Follow the same advice in treating them. Naturally, you'll have to work on the appropriate sets of muscles when you start exercising to get back flexibility and strength.

QUADRICEPS

Quadriceps muscle pulls are not common sports injuries, but when one does occur it can be disabling. Running hard backward or jumping suddenly is usually the cause. Too much stress on a tight muscle produces a sudden tearing in it. The pain is immediate and you know you are done for the day. Since the quadriceps is such a large muscle, only a portion of it tears. You can still straighten your knee and lift your leg, but the effort hurts.

Such tears generally take place in the rectus femoris, located near the middle of the four-part quadriceps muscle. If only a few fibers are torn, rest will heal them. If the tear is complete, it may have to be repaired by surgery. A complete tear generally leaves a hole or defect in the muscle, with a bulge of muscle above it which you probably will be able to feel. Since muscles normally are under tension, after being torn they retract or shorten. If you have normal strength, most surgeons won't repair a torn muscle since that is so hard to do. Tear apart a piece of fresh steak and see how easy it is to sew *that* together.

You can prevent this kind of tearing by keeping your quadriceps both flexible and strong. If it happens to you, use ice and an elastic wrap. If the injury is severe, you may need crutches for a few days. Don't try to play any sport until the pain is entirely gone, you can freely bend your knee and you've recovered normal flexibility and strength. This may take six weeks. If you push back too soon, all you'll do is hurt yourself again.

THIGH BRUISE

A thigh bruise is a hematoma of the quadriceps muscle. It can be a serious injury, maybe keeping an athlete out of commission for the entire season. The massive collection of blood in the muscle is painful and severely restricts your ability to bend your knee. Your strength, of course, is limited. Ice and compression plus rest are necessary for healing. You have to restore full flexibility and strength before competing again. Injuries of this kind are sometimes complicated by bone being laid down in the hematoma—a condition called myositis ossificans, which really prolongs the recovery period.

HIPS

Hip problems are not very common with athletes, and it's a good thing because the joint is quite large and complex, surrounded by muscles, tendons, ligaments and a variety of other vulnerable body mechanisms.

HIP TENDINITIS

The gluteus medius, the large strong muscle that runs from the rim of the pelvis to the top of the femur, is the one that allows you to stand on one leg. Repeated lateral shifts and twists of the hips and trunk may cause microscopic tearing of the tendon attachment and lead to tendinitis. As in all other tendinitis, ice, aspirin, activity based on the symptoms and your own patience will eventually give you relief.

The pain of hip tendinitis is worse when you stand on one leg, or go up and down stairs, and sometimes also when you lie on the affected side at night. You can often find a tender spot if you push over the point of your hip. If you get too uncomfortable, see a doctor.

HIP JOINT

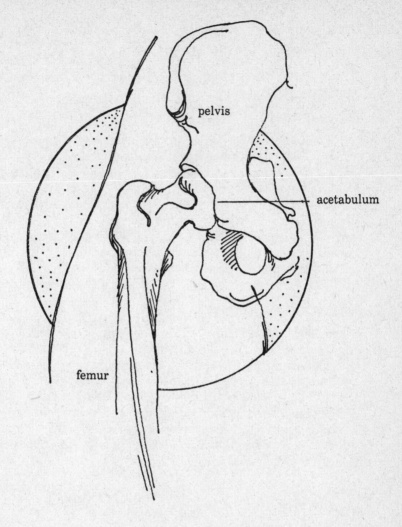

The stretching exercises described in Chapter 14 should reduce the risk of getting this kind of tendinitis.

HIP POINTER

This is a condition you hear mentioned in the sports pages from time to time. It is a bruise of the iliac crest—the rim of the pelvis that you can feel as a definite hard point just beneath the skin. It can be extremely painful, and may keep an athlete out of play for a week or more. Like all bruises, it has to heal by itself. You can treat the symptoms with ice.

THE HAND

You can hurt your intricately structured hands in playing most any sport, but there are two common injuries that seem to beat out all the others: jammed fingers and mallet finger. In Chapter 11, on bicycling, we've indicated some other kinds of hand problems that cyclists need to come to grips with.

JAMMED FINGERS

Fingers jammed in the line of play seem to be a necessary evil for athletes. They occur when a ball is caught (or not caught) on the end of a finger. Jammed fingers aren't usually serious. They hurt, swell, turn black and blue, won't move right and may take a long time, as much as six months, to heal completely. Ice and taping the injured finger against the one next to it will usually allow you to continue to play once the pain subsides. Taping helps prevent getting hurt again. If you have a lot of pain or disability, or if you see any deformity, go to a doctor for treatment. Don't let some nonprofessional pull a dislocated finger back into joint for you. That could make the situation worse.

BASEBALL OR MALLET FINGER

Baseball or mallet finger is a more serious problem. It occurs the same way but involves the distal joint, at the tip of the finger. Either the extensor tendon of the finger is torn from its attachment to bone or the bone itself is broken away. In either case the tip of the finger droops and cannot be actively straightened. This injury needs to be treated by a physician. The finger should be splinted in extension for six weeks. Keep the splint on constantly for the entire six weeks. If you allow the finger to droop once, the effect of the splint is ruined and you may end up with a permanent droop.

THE ELBOW

Elbow problems are caused mainly by overuse. Whether you're a tennis player, golfer or pitcher, chances are you haven't gotten your forearm muscles in shape to do the things you ask of your elbow. Both strength and flexibility are necessary to keep you out of trouble.

TENNIS ELBOW

We've talked about tennis elbow in connection with racquet sports, since that is mainly where it is a problem. Golfers can get it too, on either side of the elbow. This tendinitis is a self-limiting problem that will eventually heal itself if you can put up with it. Good strength, flexibility and technique prevent it. Ice relieves it. The rest of the details are in Chapter 13.

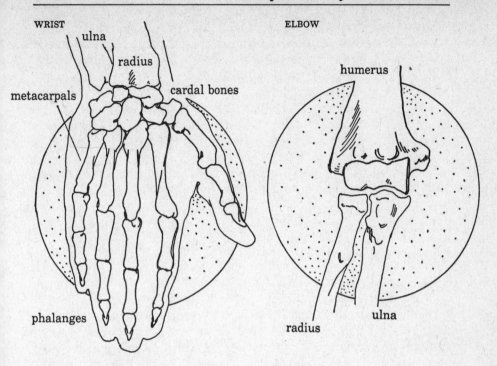

WRIST

ulna

radius

metacarpals

cardal bones

phalanges

ELBOW

humerus

radius

ulna

LITTLE LEAGUE ELBOW

Throwing a ball places a great deal of stress on the arm. The throwing elbow of a professional pitcher eventually wears out. Sandy Koufax had to put his arm in an ice bath after every game to relieve the pain. Surgery gave him an extra couple of years, but the trouble finally forced him to retire. Almost every major league pitcher is unable to straighten his arm fully. This is due either to arthritis or to contracture of the elbow. This contracture or tightening of the capsule of the elbow joint is probably caused by overuse or chronic irritation. Both problems are evidence of the severe stresses applied to the elbow. Little League elbow may sound like kid's stuff, but it's a serious problem that can destroy the career of a major leaguer, or do enough damage to a youngster to knock him out of sports competition for the rest of his life. It is certainly not one of those conditions you can ignore and hope it will get better.

Little League elbow can mean one of two things. The first is a problem on the inside of the elbow, where the flexor muscles of the hand and wrist attach. Tendinitis at this attachment follows repeated small tears due to overuse. In more severe cases a piece of bone may be pulled away at the attachment, the medial epicondyle. The tendinitis should heal with time. If a piece of bone has been pulled away, the injury is usually permanent.

The other problem occurs on the outside of the elbow and involves damage to the joint surfaces of the humerus and radius. In severe cases a loose chip that has broken off the surface of either bone, usually the humerus, produces pain and inability to straighten the arm. Sports doctors used to think that throwing curve balls too early was the cause of Little League elbow. Now most of them believe that throwing any pitch too hard, too often, is the cause. Little League officials are attempting to solve the problem by limiting the number of pitches a youngster is permitted to throw in a week.

If a youngster has persistent elbow pain, something is abnormal. Stop pitching and see an orthopedic surgeon.

SHOULDERS

SHOULDER TENDINITIS

The older we get, the tighter we get. This is why so many recreational athletes have problems with shoulder tendinitis. In most of the things we do in normal living, our arms hang at our sides or are raised no more than shoulder high. Doing anything that repeatedly requires the shoulders to be stretched into an abnormal position may be asking for trouble. Throwing a baseball, serving a tennis ball, swinging a golf club and swimming all put the arms high over the head and even behind it. If we don't work to restore some flexibility first, those tight muscles and tendons may tear when forced into abnormal positions. Many small tears produce scar tissue, which is painful when stretched. This thickened scar tissue may also be pinched between the head of the humerus and the acromion. In either instance, pain is the result. It can be a sharp jab when you move, or a truly agonizing one that prevents you from moving the arm at all. Lying on the shoulder at night is usually painful, too.

Ice and aspirin should be used to relieve the pain if it is minor. If it becomes so severe that you can get no relief, see a doctor. This is one place where a shot of hydrocortisone often gives dramatic relief.

Of course, the best treatment of shoulder tendinitis is prevention. It is really quite simple to keep your shoulder muscles flexible all during the year. The exercises are in Chapter 4. Do them daily, and especially right before you play.

ROTATOR CUFF TEARS

Occasionally people suffer major tearing of the rotator cuff tendons of the shoulder, whose function is to help stabilize the shoulder as it is moved. Such injuries occur when you fall against the ground or a wall. Being of sound mind, you put your arm out to protect yourself. If you land on the side of the elbow and all the muscles are contracted to

SHOULDER

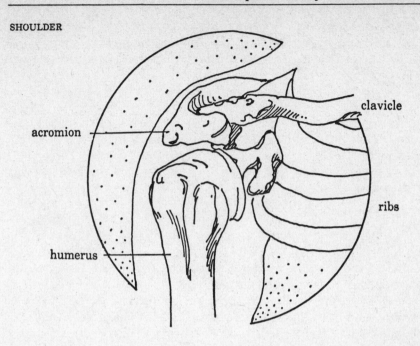

acromion

humerus

clavicle

ribs

break the fall, the rotator cuff tendons may tear, especially if they are tight and inflexible. You'll have pain and trouble in lifting your arm above your head and in rotating your shoulder. If the tear is large, you may even have trouble moving your arm away from your side. See a doctor if the pain doesn't subside in a few days after a fall like this. You may need an arthrogram to make the diagnosis. Such tears should be repaired in young, active people—which you are if you're an athlete, no matter what your age.

SHOULDER SEPARATION

A shoulder separation can occur when you dive for a ball and land on the point of your shoulder. The shoulder bones are driven down, and the ligaments that hold the clavicle in place against the acromion are torn. If the tear is complete, the clavicle pops up as a prominence at the top of the shoulder. If the tear is incomplete, shoulder motion is painful and you'll find a tender spot on the top of the shoulder. You should seek medical advice about a shoulder separation.

SHOULDER DISLOCATIONS

If a lot of force is applied to your arm when it is up and back, your shoulder may be popped out of joint or dislocated. This hurts, and you will have no doubt that something serious has happened. If you think you might have dislocated your shoulder, there's a simple test you can do to find out. If you can put your hand on your opposite shoulder, and your elbow against your chest, the shoulder is not out of joint.

A dislocation at any joint is an emergency. Nerves and arteries are usually closest and most firmly attached to bone right at the joint. If the bones are out of place, the nerves and vessels will be stretched and may be permanently damaged unless the dislocation is reduced promptly. After reduction, a dislocated shoulder should be immobilized completely for three weeks. Keep your bandages on and keep the shoulder still. If you move the shoulder too soon, you won't have allowed sufficient healing and run the risk of chronic problems with dislocation.

CLAVICLE FRACTURE

Falling and trying to brace yourself can break your collarbone. The clavicle is one of the first bones to ossify, and thus one of the most brittle. If there is a fracture, you can usually find a tender spot over the bone and feel the two fragments move. Strapping your arm to your side will make the trip to the hospital more comfortable.

Clavicle fractures almost always heal in six weeks. As soon as the pain subsides your doctor should start you on some exercises so that the shoulder won't tighten up too much.

THE BACK

Any sport, in fact any*thing,* can cause an aching, injured back. Most low back pain is really a posture problem. Consider the trunk as a cylinder. The spine is the back wall, the abdominal muscles are the front wall. If the front wall is weak and balloons out, the whole cylinder is weakened, so that when extra stress is applied to the back wall, the result is back pain.

Twisting, turning, jumping, arching of the back and the repeated jolts of running are part of every sport. If the muscles of the trunk are too weak to support the back properly, there is going to be trouble. Certainly there are other problems that can contribute to backache, such as congenital abnormalities, disc degeneration, arthritis or a slipped disc, but all of these are made worse by weak muscles and better by strong ones.

SCIATICA

This is a pain down the back of the leg caused by irritation of the sciatic nerve. It can sometimes be confused with a hamstring injury, especially in runners. If the pain is associated with backache or came on insidiously rather than suddenly, the chances are that it's sciatica. Most often sciatica is due to a slipped disc. The discs act somewhat in the manner of shock absorbers between the vertebrae. If a disc wears out or degenerates, it may bulge and press against a nerve root where it branches off the spinal cord. The result will be sciatica.

Back pain and sciatica are both usually aggravated by sitting, standing or walking, and relieved by lying down. With sciatica you may notice some numbness in your leg or foot. Coughing, sneezing and straining to move your bowels may make it hurt more. Back pain is usually aggravated by moving and may be a sharp jab. Sciatica feels like a bolt of electricity or a burning sensation down your leg.

If you are in trouble of this kind, lie down; sitting won't help you much. You've got to get the weight of your upper trunk off your lower back. Bed rest is the cure for backache. Aspirin may help the pain somewhat. Heat is soothing and feels good, but most people with back pain parboil themselves. Even though a little heat is good, a lot of it is not better. Most of the pain comes from swelling around the muscles and joints of your back, and heat tends to cause more swelling. Too much will make it worse. Use a heating pad on the lowest setting for 15 or 20 minutes at a time. Don't use it more than 4 times a day and *don't* sleep with it on.

If a week or ten days of bed rest doesn't give you relief, or if the pain becomes really intense, see your doctor. You should also see a doctor if you notice increasing numbness in your leg while you're staying in bed. And if you develop any weakness in your leg, that's a sign of a more serious problem and you belong in a hospital.

If you do end up in a hospital, the treatment will usually be the same: more bed rest. Once you've started to improve, you'll begin doing exercises to rehabilitate your muscles. If you fail to improve, surgery may be necessary. Fortunately, this isn't often the case. About 90 percent of slipped discs get well with rest.

The majority of back pain is preventable. That's *your* responsibility—not your doctor's. Time lost from work as a result of back pain runs into millions of dollars annually. Weak abdominal muscles and tight back and hamstring muscles are major causes. Prevention calls for daily work on strengthening abdominal muscles and on making hamstrings and trunk flexible. If you have a history of back pain, you will have to make a commitment to becoming fit. You'll have to get enthusiastic about your daily exercise routine.

Some sports just aren't for some people. Running, with the repeated pounding that is transmitted from your legs to your back, can aggravate back problems. If you have them, a switch to swimming or cycling as a fitness program may be called for.

SPONDYLOLISTHESIS

Another cause of back pain is spondylolisthesis. Doctors used to think it was a congenital problem, but now believe that it is due to a stress fracture of the bony arch that is a part of each vertebra. This bony arch, which protects the spinal cord and the nerve roots, is attached to the back side of each vertebra. It helps to keep the spine in line and to prevent it from arching too far. If there is a defect in the arch, one vertebra may slide forward on the one below it. The result is pain in the back and sometimes down both legs. Most people with this problem have extremely tight hamstrings. The problem is seen frequently in interior linemen, among football players, and in volleyball players who dive to retrieve balls.

If bed rest and exercises don't give relief from the pain, or there are repeated bouts of it, a spinal fusion may be necessary.

NECK INJURIES

Almost everyone at some time or other ends up with a crick. Arthritis of the cervical spine—which you may feel as a crick in the neck—is almost a universal problem. Forty-five out of fifty people over the age of 50, when X-rays are taken, show changes consistent with arthritis. Many of these people may never have had symptoms, but most eventually will. Poor posture and weak neck muscles are generally responsible for the trouble.

The symptom of cervical spine arthritis is pain—most often in the neck, but it may also be felt along the shoulder blade and down the arm. The pain is made worse by turning the head and just by being upright. There may be numbness in the arms when the pain is severe. Sometimes it is difficult to decide where the pain that runs along the arm is coming from. Is it your shoulder or your neck? If it's the former, shoulder motion will make it hurt more; if it's the latter, neck motion will aggravate it.

As with back pain, the treatment for neck pain is rest. Since your head weighs 12 or 13 pounds, you need to get the stress of that weight off your neck. If you sprain your wrist, you don't walk around holding up a bowling ball all day. The same principle applies to your neck. Lie down. That's the only way you can rest what hurts.

Fortunately, very few neck problems occur in sports. Those that do occur are in collision sports such as soccer and football, or in connection with falls, as on a trampoline or in a diving accident.

If a neck injury occurs in sports it should be treated as a potentially serious problem. Don't touch or move the injured person. Let the problem be handled by someone who knows what to do. This is a true emergency. Get help.

HEAD INJURIES

Minor cuts, bumps and bruises of the head are common occurrences in sports. Significant lacerations need to be sutured; the bumps and bruises can usually be ignored, though they should be treated with ice.

Occasionally, major head injuries take place in sports. Any loss of consciousness is potentially serious. The injured player should be transported to a hospital for observation. One who is unconscious must be handled as if there were a neck injury that could cause paralysis. Get expert help before moving that person.

EYE INJURIES

Eye injuries can cause blindness. Anyone suffering such an injury in sports should be examined by a physician.

More and more injuries are happening in racquet sports. The most important thing you can do is prevent them. Safety glasses are helpful, and sports goggles are now available and should be worn by every racquetball player. They can be ground to your prescription, and the new models give you wide-angle vision without distortion. They are your best protection.

THE MOST COMMON INJURIES, LISTED IN ORDER OF FREQUENCY

Running
1. Knee
2. Achilles tendon
3. Shin splints
4. Arch
5. Heel

Swimming
1. Shoulder
2. Knee

Cycling
1. Knee
2. Hands
3. Calf
4. Back

Skiing
1. Knee
2. Shoulder
3. Ankle
4. Back
5. Lower leg

Racquet Sports
1. Elbow
2. Calf
3. Shoulder
4. Ankle

Golf
1. Back
2. Elbow
3. Shoulder

Bat and ball
1. Ankle
2. Hamstrings
3. Hands
4. Elbow
5. Shoulder

Basketball, volleyball
1. Ankle
2. Hands
3. Knee
4. Calf
5. Foot

Soccer, football
1. Knee
2. Hamstrings
3. Groin
4. Hands
5. Ankle

HOT SPOTS: FIND YOUR SPORT, SPOT THE MOST COMMON INJURIES

Every sport carries some risk. The more you understand the risks, the better off you are. We've listed some of the most common injury sites for some of the most common sports. Find your sport, spot your problem area, and you'll find helpful information about injury treatment and prevention in the pages indicated alongside each body part.

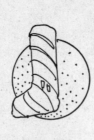

	Foot, heel p. 233	Ankle p. 237	Lower leg pp. 104, 143, 239	Knee p. 241	Hamstring pp. 110, 137, 250
Running	X	X	X	X	X
Swimming				X	
Cycling		X		X	X
Skiing		X	X	X	X
Racquet sports	X				X
Golf					
Bat and ball	X	X		X	X
Basketball, volleyball		X	X	X	X
Football, soccer	X	X		X	X

	Groin pp. 117, 251	Quadriceps pp. 108, 135, 251	Hips p. 252	Hand p. 254	Elbow pp. 120, 254
Running	X	X	X		
Swimming					
Cycling				X	X
Skiing	X	X		X	X
Racquet sports				X	X
Golf			X	X	X
Bat and ball	X	X		X	
Basketball, volleyball	X	X		X	
Football, soccer	X	X		X	

	Shoulder pp. 119, 148, 256	Back pp. 148, 258	Neck p. 260	Head p. 260	Eye p. 261
Running	X	X			
Swimming					X
Cycling		X	X		
Skiing	X			X	
Racquet sports	X			X	X
Golf	X	X			
Bat and ball	X			X	
Basketball, volleyball	X	X	X	X	
Football, soccer	X	X	X	X	

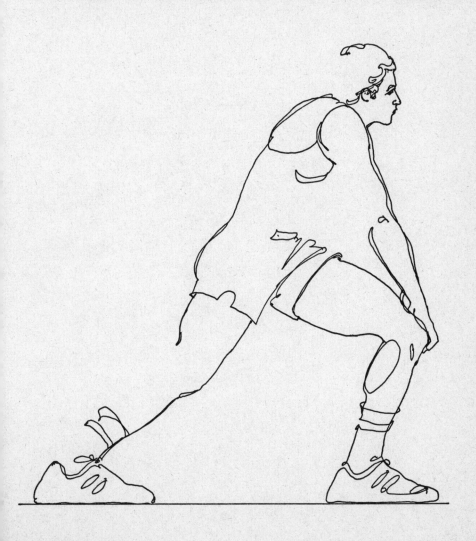

17. Glossary of Sports

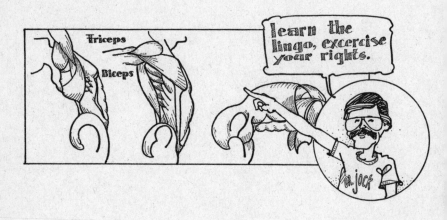

Medicine Terms

Every science, business or field of technology has its own vocabulary, its own special jargon. This is as true for bankers and piano tuners as it is for boiler repairmen and doctors. Special words, computer printouts, Latin names, unfamiliar technical phrases may make communication *within* the medical field easier, but it can make communication *from* the medical field much more difficult to understand than if the doctor simply spoke plain American English.

Some doctors take the time to do just that, but most don't. Or can't. So, more often than not, patients are lost in a fog when it comes to what their injury is, how it's best treated and how best to prevent it from happening again.

If you could get past the technical terms, see through the mystique of medicine that is practiced on you and really come to grips with your problem, you would be a much happier, healthier patient. One way to do that is to try and learn the language.

Being more responsible for your own health means not accepting a diagnosis, such as a torn meniscus in your acromio-clavicular joint, without a full explanation first. See your injury in context and ask your doctor questions. Where is it? How could it have happened? What can I do to prevent it from happening again? It's reasonable to expect your doctor to speak *your* language, but just in case he doesn't, you'll do well to learn a little of his. That's what this glossary is for.

Here, some of the most common terms used in sports medicine are explained. Muscles are listed separately, at the end.

ABRASION—When you fall down and scrape away the outer layer of skin cells, you've got yourself an abrasion. It's usually not serious and you can take care of it yourself. Clean it with soap and water and let it heal—that's it. Salves and ointments may make you feel better, but they don't make your body heal any faster. Indeed, you're better off not spending your money on those products since they only tend to get in the way of your own natural healing process.

ACROMION—The tip of your shoulder blade; that bony prominence at the top of your shoulder.

ARTHRITIS—"Arth" is for joint, and "itis" means inflammation, so arthritis is an inflammation of a joint, any joint, such as your knee, your elbow, your wrist, etc. There are several kinds of arthritis. One is called *rheumatoid arthritis* and it is a systemic disease that cruelly affects many different joints, throughout the entire body.

The more common kind is *degenerative* or *osteoarthritis,* and this is typically what your doctor tells you you have a touch of, or are developing, in that aching knee or painful wrist. This kind of arthritis is a natural effect of aging and use—sort of like gray hair of the joint.

The joint's surface—your doctor calls it the articular cartilage—begins to wear away, and then you're left with inflammation and pain. The inflammation is caused at least partially by small pieces of this chipped, damaged articular surface that float about in the joint and irritate the joint lining.

Why some older folks are crippled by degenerative arthritis, while others may live a long time with only mild discomfort, is still something of a mystery to us.

We do know that an insult or an injury to the joint surface—and that can happen in sports or from an improper rehabilitation program—may accelerate the wearing-down process and cause a *traumatic arthritis,* which is really a form of degenerative arthritis.

There's no clear-cut, all-purpose answer to questions about the compatibility of arthritis and athletics. We're not even sure at this point what effect long-distance running will have on runners' knees 10 or 20 years down the road. Major league pitchers are sure to get arthritis in the elbow from all the wear and tear put on their throwing arm, and we can't be absolutely sure that running 40, 60 or 100 miles a week every week for years won't speed up the natural degenerative process.

Generally speaking, if you've got arthritis, you shouldn't be involved in sports that will cause undue stress and strain on the already-injured joint. Of course, there are exceptions. Dedicated athletes determined to continue playing tennis, or running, or skiing may be willing to risk damage, because they can't see giving up their fun. A fitness sport like swimming can be fun too, and it is ideal for people with arthritis since it lets the joints move freely, with minimum pain and pressure.

ARTHROGRAM—Many sports injuries require an arthrogram for proper diagnosis. In the fall of 1979, it cost approximately $130 (the way X-ray prices are going up, we ought to include the month, too), and can be done by a radiologist or orthopedist in a hospital or specially equipped doctor's office. It's a series of X-rays taken of a joint (usually the knee) in all different positions. Air and/or dye is injected into the joint to act as a contrast medium, which allows the doctor to tell whether or not your sports injury caused your cartilage to tear. Your doctor can't tell that from a routine X-ray and he needs to know because treatment will vary; a strained patellar tendon will heal itself but a torn cartilage is best remedied with surgery. Nature abhors a vacuum, and joints can't tolerate loose ends.

ARTHROSCOPE—This is a relatively new procedure in medicine, and a handy diagnostic tool. Determining what is really causing joint pain, especially knee pain, can be tough because it's a complicated system and many things could be at fault. Thanks to the development of fiber-optic light sources, doctors can now look into an ailing joint and see more of the structure than they've ever seen before, even during actual surgery. The instrument is inserted directly into the joint (with the patient asleep or under a local anesthetic), and some surgeons are even operating through tiny instruments adapted for the arthroscope so that no large incision is required. That's still in the experimental stage, though.

BURSA—The bursa is a protective sac over bony prominences that helps the skin or muscle slide over them. If something bad happens to one of your bursa, you've got bursitis, an inflammation of the bursa.

It most commonly occurs to athletes who play sports that require them to repeatedly raise their arms and shoulders, like tennis, racquetball, swimming, baseball, etc. A fall or a blow can cause the bursa to fill with blood, but usually bursitis is due to chronic irritation and the sac is filled with a clear, yellow fluid. When the bursa is inflamed, the wall becomes thickened and it may feel as if there are loose bodies floating around inside the sac.

Racquet sport players tend to aggravate the *olecranon bursa* over the point of their elbow, and another common one that causes a lot of pain in the shoulder area is an inflammation of the *subdeltoid bursa,* under the deltoid muscle at the shoulder. Proper warm-up and strengthening exercises will help prevent bursitis, but once you've got it, you treat it like tendinitis or any other kind of inflammation.

CALCANEUS—Your heel bone.

CARTILAGE—Cartilage is the gristle, the tough, white connective tissue in the joints, and it is frequently involved in sports injuries of every description.

There are two kinds of cartilage. The *articular cartilage* is the firm, shining joint surface (made up of hyaline cartilage) and every joint has some. It helps joint surfaces slide on each other.

The second, most commonly discussed cartilage, is the *semilunar cartilage,* or meniscus. It's in the knee and most often causes problems there, but a meniscus may also be present in your wrist, or your *acromio-clavicular* joint (the joint between the collarbone and the scapula) and your *temporo-mandibular* joint (the jaw).

This kind of cartilage is made up of fibrocartilage, as opposed to hyaline cartilage. It is softer and more flexible than hard, white hyaline cartilage. The meniscus is in the knee joint to help stabilize it. If you tear your cartilage in a fall or sports accident, you are left with a damaged knee, and an uneven surface inside the joint that can injure the joint unless it is removed. Since this cartilage has no blood supply, it can't heal itself. That's why most doctors will recommend surgery. If you work hard to rehabilitate your knee after your operation, you should be able to return to sports in a minimum of six weeks.

CHONDROMALACIA—This refers to the roughening of the undersurface of the patella, or kneecap. It is another common sore spot in sports, particularly running, and causes considerable knee pain. It is a form of degenerative arthritis, and though we're not always sure why it happens, experience has shown that bent-knee, weight-bearing work, such as squatting, climbing stairs or hills, and improper strengthening exercises, will aggravate the condition. Treatment has to be individualized for each patient.

CLAVICLE—Your collarbone.

CONTUSION—A bruise from a blow, or a fall, or maybe a misguided racquetball. What happens is blood vessels rupture, and their bloody contents spill and accumulate under the skin. Since our skin is translucent, we can see the discoloration: a fresh bruise shows up reddish-blue; an older bruise is yellow-green. The colors change as the blood pigment breaks up and eventually is removed. Bruises will heal by themselves and rarely are they anything to worry about.

EXTENSION—Straightening a joint, as opposed to flexion, which is bending a joint. Most exercises are combinations of the two.

FEMUR—Your thigh bone. It's big; if you press anywhere above your knee, you can't miss it.

FIBULA—The smaller of the two lower leg bones.

FLEXION—Bending a joint, as opposed to extension, which is straightening a joint. Most exercises are a combination of the two.

FRACTURE—A fracture is any kind of disruption in the overall integrity of the bone. Fractures can occur following any collision, whether it is with your opponent, teammate, the ground or any other immovable object. They always require professional treatment. Fractures hurt when they happen and continue to hurt afterward. They may be accompanied by a snap or a crack. They usually continue to hurt more when you attempt to move. That part doesn't get better. You may feel a sense of instability, as though something isn't connected correctly. You can usually find a tender point if you push where it hurts and if you push hard enough you can often feel some crackling, called *crepitus*. Most of the time you won't be all that anxious to do this, though. If you see any deformity, anything out of line, you don't have to know much else to know that you are in trouble. Almost always, when there has been a fracture, you'll know that something serious has occurred. You may be nauseated. If so, don't worry about that; it's a normal reaction.

If you suspect that you have a broken bone, don't move or let anyone try to move you until some kind of splint has been applied. Motion of the fractured part will cause more pain and may damage nerves or blood vessels, or even cause the bone fragments to poke through the skin. This makes a serious injury potentially disastrous. If there is an open wound, the chance of infection increases. This is a true emergency which calls for prompt surgery.

HEMATOMA—A big bruise, sometimes a lump, that comes from an injury, a fall or something else unexpected, like a hard-hit tennis ball. As with a bruise, the blood vessels are broken and the hematoma that results is really just the collection of blood in the tissues. In time, the body will absorb the damaged goods, but you can help matters somewhat with ice and compression with an elastic bandage to help limit the bleeding. A bruise is superficial but a hematoma can be serious and should be watched.

HUMERUS—The upper arm bone.

ISOMETRIC/ISOKINETIC/ISOTONIC EXERCISES—These are three kinds of weight-resistance exercises designed to strengthen muscles. In isometrics, the muscle sustains a maximum contraction but it does not move. In isokinetics, the muscle is working against a variable resistance at a constant speed. In isotonic exercise, the muscle lifts a resistance (a weight) through a wide range of motion. All three kinds of exercise have their advantages and their disadvantages in terms of strengthening and rehabilitating weak muscles. More details in Chapter 8.

LACERATION—A disruption in the integrity of the skin, or, in plain English, a cut. Deep cuts may require stitches and a doctor, but most will heal all by themselves if you just wash it and leave it alone. Salves and bandages don't really help and may, in fact, hinder the natural healing process.

LIGAMENT—This is tissue which connects bone to bone. For instance, the *medial collateral ligament* connects the femur to the tibia on the inside of your knee.

METACARPALS—The five hand bones.

METATARSALS—The five forefoot bones.

RADIUS—The forearm bone on the thumb side.

SCAPULA—Your shoulder blade.

SPRAIN—A tear in a ligament, any ligament, but in sports injuries it frequently happens in the ankle. A fall can cause it, and so can a sudden twist. You can get a partial tear or a complete tear; both cause swelling and pain. A complete tear or a severe sprain may require surgical repair. A moderate sprain may require immobilization (a cast) until it heals, so it won't become a complete rip. A mild sprain with only a few fibers torn usually can be self-treated, with some ice and a little rest.

STRAIN—Any tear in a muscle or a tendon is called a strain. Like a sprain, it can happen after a sudden injury, but most often athletes bring on their strains with too much use and too little flexibility. Tendon tears require surgery in most cases, even if the tear is incomplete. Muscle tears are almost always incomplete, and they rarely require surgery.

STRESS FRACTURE—This is a small, hairline crack in one wall or cortex of a bone. It's an incomplete fracture and it is increasingly common among runners, sometimes called a fatigue fracture. It usually comes from overuse, too much pounding. Symptoms are pain, swelling, redness and the fracture itself may not show up on an X-ray until two or three weeks after the symptoms appear. The metatarsal bones and the tibia are the ones most often involved. The treatment is rest until it heals (six weeks) and it rarely needs a cast.

SYNOVITIS and SYNOVIUM—The synovium is the joint lining. Its function is to secrete joint fluid which lubricates your joint and makes motion possible. When the lining gets inflamed, it's called synovitis. Many things can irritate the joint lining: a blow that causes bleeding, particles of articular cartilage in arthritis, a torn cartilage, bacteria, etc. An irritated lining responds by producing too much joint fluid and that's called *effusion*. It's also called water on the knee when it happens to that joint, though it could happen anywhere. Almost every knee injury involves some fluid in the joint, which the doctor can remove with a needle and syringe called aspiration. The problem comes in diagnosing what caused the fluid. Your doctor ought to treat the cause, not just the effect, the effusion.

TALUS—This is the top bone of the foot. Along with the end of the tibia and fibula, it makes up the ankle joint.

TENDON and TENDINITIS—This is probably the most common chronic problem for all recreational athletes. The tendon is the fibrous connective tissue that attaches all of your muscles to all of your bones. When it gets inflamed, it's called tendinitis. Why it gets inflamed is not 100 percent clear, but most likely it is an overuse syndrome—too much stress on the tendon with too little flexibility. If you work out without stretching out first, you can cause many tiny tears in the tendon tissue. You won't feel it and these microscopic tears will heal, but that's not the end of it. When the tears heal, they leave scar tissue and next time you run, or ski, or leap after that forehand smash, you may rip the scar tissue. And that really hurts. Tendinitis is a self-limiting disease, meaning it will go away by itself. In time, the body will replace the scar tissue with normal, healthy tendon tissue. But it takes a long time, and the process can be painful. You can use ice and elastic bandages to help cut down pain and swelling, and your doctor may help matters somewhat with anti-inflammatory drugs or even a shot of cortisone. You're best off, though, just letting it heal by itself. In the meantime, you can continue your sport as long as you can deal with the pain. See Chapter 4 for more details.

TIBIA—The larger of the two lower leg bones.

ULNA—The forearm bone, opposite side from thumb.

MAJOR MUSCLES

BICEPS—The upper arm muscles that bend the elbow.

TRICEPS—The upper arm muscles that extend the elbow.

QUADRICEPS—The anterior thigh muscles (directly above the knee) that extend the knee.

HAMSTRINGS—The posterior thigh muscles that flex the knee.

GASTROCNEMIUS and SOLEUS—These two together are called the TRICEPS SURAE and they form your calf muscle.

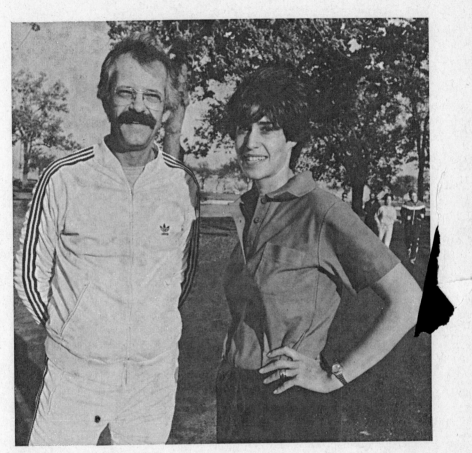

ABOUT THE AUTHORS

Dr. David Bachman is director of the Center for Sports Medicine at Northwestern University Medical School. He is an orthopedic surgeon and team doctor for the Chicago Bull's basketball team and the women's pro basketball team, the Hustle. Marilynn Preston is a feature writer for the *Chicago Tribune* and created the nationally-syndicated column, "Dr. Jock."